M000235356

"'Expect the unexpected,' Jerry Sargeant states in his book *Healing with Light Frequencies*, and I sincerely invite you to do just that. In his vision and approach of healing, the author moves way beyond what many people may see as possible during treatments. As a result, he encourages the individual to explore and embody his or her full healing potential as well as the full potential as an incarnated human being."

— TJITZE DE JONG, Brennan Healing Science practitioner
and author of *Energetic Cellular Healing and Cancer*

"There are many people who have written books on self-healing, but there are very few indeed who introduce the subject area of quantum energy—the field and how to access it. Fewer still who show you, once there, how to create verifiable results in the physical world. In his book *Healing with Light Frequencies* Jerry does just this. He goes into great depth, showing you how to interact with this wonderful space and how you can use the quantum world to instigate incredible life changes. I have used Jerry's tools and techniques and have seen amazing results. Results that have had others saying, 'Wow! What did you just do?' Jerry has turned what is a complex subject into child's play. It's fun and exciting. It's pure genius."

— KIM HUMPHRIES, pharmacist

"As a doctor I am aware of the medical field's limitations. I was searching for answers, and *Healing with Light Frequencies* gave me insights on healing techniques that are very powerful and have produced remarkable clinical results. During a healing session with a stroke victim suffering from paralysis, my colleagues and I could see visible effects. The cells, tissues, and organs each produced certain collective frequencies when working with the light frequencies of Star Magic. All levels of the mind and body achieved rapid shifts. Star Magic has enabled me to heal with no medication and no referral for surgery. Everything healed using the energy of Star Magic and the tools within *Healing with Light Frequencies*. What I achieved as a doctor using Star Magic were fast, physical, and verifiable results. Thank you, Jerry Sargeant, for the amazing teachings and this life-changing book."

— DR. VANDANA RANNJJIT ASHAR, B.H.M.S. (Homeopathic Medical Science),
Access Body Process facilitator and energy healer

HEALING WITH LIGHT FREQUENCIES

THE TRANSFORMATIVE POWER OF STAR MAGIC

JERRY SARGEANT

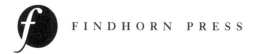

FINDHORN PRESS

Findhorn Press
One Park Street
Rochester, Vermont 05767
www.findhornpress.com

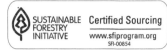

Text stock is SFI certified

Findhorn Press is a division of Inner Traditions International

Originally published in 2016 by Findhorn Press under the title *Star Magic: Heal the YOU-Niverse*

Disclaimer
The information in this book is given in good faith and is neither intended to diagnose any physical or mental condition nor to serve as a substitute for informed medical advice or care. Please contact your health professional for medical advice and treatment. Neither author nor publisher can be held liable by any person for any loss or damage whatsoever which may arise from the use of this book or any of the information therein.

Cataloging-in-Publication data for this title is available from the Library of Congress

ISBN 978-1-64411-109-3 (print)
ISBN 978-1-64411-110-9 (ebook)

Printed and bound in the United States by Lake Book Manufacturing, Inc.
The text stock is SFI certified. The Sustainable Forestry Initiative® program promotes sustainable forest management.

10 9 8 7 6 5 4 3

Edited by Michael Hawkins
Illustrations by Emma Walters, Aran-Sarah Sweetmore (p. 102), Damian Keenan (p. 247)
Text design and layout by Damian Keenan
This book was typeset in Adobe Garamond Pro, Calluna Sans and Museo with ITC Century Std Book Condensed used as a display typeface.

To send correspondence to the author of this book, mail a first-class letter to the author c/o Inner Traditions • Bear & Company, One Park Street, Rochester, VT 05767, USA and we will forward the communication, or contact the author directly at **www.starmagichealing.com**

Contents

I am not a healer, I am but just a shell.
My spirit friends work through me to help make people well.
They use me as a channel, their healing gifts to pour,
into the bodies of needy folk, I'm a channel nothing more.
Please don't call me a healer, I'm no different from you,
I just give my time to serve God, and see what I can do.
To help the spirit brethren, pass on their healing balm,
and pray that folks I meet each day experience no harm.
Please don't call me a healer, my hands are nothing new,
I am just like an instrument to help folks such as you.
And when my time approaches for this earthly frame to die,
my soul will cry out thank you God for using such as I.

Introduction

How many self-help books have you read? How many seminars have you been to? What are you looking for? What is it that keeps you searching? Do you think it's actually possible to find what you are looking for?

If you believe this book may contain the answers you so desperately desire, then I strongly suggest you put it back down. If, however you are ready and willing to saddle up, and take a journey with me, through space, and the dimensional doorway that allows us to ride the inter-planetary waves of our beloved Cosmos, then buy it and e x p e r i e n c e it.

If you are ready to leave behind everything that you have ever known, been taught or made to believe was real, and be swallowed up by a world that knows no logic, yet makes perfect intuitive sense, and open the channels of communication with Ancient Civilizations, our beloved allies of the Spirit World, who guide me day-in day-out to perform distance healing, and incredible feats of psychic surgery, then sit back and ride the rhythm and vibration of time, sound and energy.

Energy never dies (END). Ancient Civilizations are not gone or dead. They are there in the mystical realm of alternate realities, waiting for our re-birth as a planet, so we can unite once more and share these Earthly planes. I use a way (not method or system) of healing that we are all capable of discovering and this book will guide you to remember. I will open my heart to you and share with you what I know and don't know, what I have remembered, by journeying though time and space, in worlds beyond ours. I was fortunate enough to have a trusted team of guides, brothers and sisters of light who ignited DNA strands deep within me, after a serious road traffic accident. They helped me remember Star Magic. I am now going to share it with you so you can unlock the true wisdom that lies in the mine of your soul.

Star Magic works at a level of super-consciousness. You cannot understand it by thinking. If you try and believe in Star Magic, it will not work for you. You must go deeper, much deeper, way down into the labyrinth of your infinite mind and the depths of your fearless heart. Here, if you are prepared to let go of the surface world, your five senses, expand your consciousness, remember all three hundred and sixty plus senses, and keep journeying, you stand a very good chance of knowing your power.

By journeying with me you will unlock your full human potential. You will know you, at a level of light and information, and begin to feel your way through life. Old paradigms will fall by the wayside as you experience a massive shift in your awareness and your abilities as a human being. That is the most extraordinary aspect of being a spiritual being, having a human experience; you get to re-discover the spiritual aspect of you. The aspect that knows no limitations, the aspect of you that can bend time and manipulate reality, that can shape-shift, bi-locate, travel inter and multi-dimensionally and be in as many places as you want at any one time.

Star Magic and Star Language will open the channels to these special gifts you have, and so much more. You will remember how to communicate telepathically, remote-view, heal yourself and the world, by raising your personal vibration and the vibration of this beautiful big blue planet Earth.

I call myself "The Facilitator" and don't take credit for what happens when I heal. The language of light and energy does the work. I have simply remembered how to direct, instruct and play with the light. I'm able to edit your Karmic Blue Print and cause huge reality shifts very quickly, with this super-charged form of healing ("Star Magic") that uses applied Quantum Physics to quickly release the physical, mental and emotional blocks/stresses/traumas that you may be experiencing, keeping you from creating and living your most extraordinary life.

The key to why this modality is so potent is that all healings happen within the inverted field and work on a deep root cellular level, and beyond – within the world of light frequencies. From this space, each one of us immediately aligns with the most authentic, whole and powerful aspect of ourselves, which in itself, creates an environment whereby profound healing takes place. This modality has been totally blowing my clients away, and is considered to be one of the most thorough and alchemizing energy healing modalities available.

Tumours, cysts, fibromyalgia, eyesight, hearts, haemorrhoids, broken bones, nervous systems, and much more have been healed. Dis-eases simply disappear as though they were never there in the first place, or mend as if by magic. I also use Star Magic to elevate business performance, remove blocks in relationships and so much more. If you're not satisfied with life you must get to know Star Magic.

Star Magic is a formula, a flexible formula but it's not a system. It's a disciplined, non-systematical way of knowing, and this formula can be adapted to suit every human being in their own special and unique way. I am going to share with you healing ways that you will not have seen before (I use the term "way" as it is expansive; a method, programme or system is rigid, with boundaries and limitations). It's not to say that no one else is using them, because they may well be. As far as I know, no one has brought the advanced Star Magic healing ways into the public arena. I experienced something similar working with Shamans in Brazil, but still, it's not the same.

I will to show you how to harness the light frequencies within individual star constellations and how each constellation matches a particular body frequency. Once the two are aligned, healing manifests. As above, so below.

The Chinese use the term Wu Wei (pronounced "oo way"), and you must live with Wu Wei to harness the full power of Star Magic. It can be translated as living in a state of spontaneous flow. You cannot try and be Wu Wei, you are it. You cannot do or become Star Magic, it flows through you. You are Star Magic. By living in a state of spontaneous flow you will harmonize with Mother Nature and vibrate at a resonant vibratory frequency that allows miracles to mould and shape your inner world, thus leaving a trail of extraordinary beauty in your outer world, a reflection of who you truly are.

I have spent months sat in Ancient Mystery Schools in Egypt, being shown, guided to remember what I had forgotten. Each morning I would wake up and spend hours in meditation, deep meditation, journeying between worlds, communicating, listening, observing and opening my brain capacity to receive intense light. Light after all is information. I will show you how you too can access this bountiful storehouse of knowledge and wisdom, held within the light and sound codes.

Deciphering these universal codes is the key. I call them Star Magic Codes of Consciousness and with them you can literally re-write the programme in someone's biological computer, their brain. I can take the old disempowering, habitual, dysfunctional software programme out, and install a new, up to date empowering one, which will serve you, your life and the planet. Every piece of information, every event; past, present and future, everything that has ever been and will ever be, is contained within each cell of your human body. *You are the YOU-Niverse.* By knowing Star Magic you will have the opportunity to re-write history now. You will see the world as a unified field of energy. A source of love with blocks hindering its natural flow. Star Magic will enable you to remove these blocks, on all levels, within and without, up above, so below, within the YOU-Niverse and so throughout the Universe, and, in turn, creating the perfect environment to heal yourself and the planet.

As you journey through these pages you will feel the information. There is magic embedded within the words, the paper, the book itself. Star Magic contains information from the Universal Database. Every human being that has ever connected with Star Magic has left something within the Star Magic Consciousness Grid that envelops this planet, something I refer to as the Star Magic Matrix. It has spread like wildfire from the moment I remembered it.

Everyone that I have ever facilitated the healing of has downloaded information on Star Magic and that information, the frequency encoded healing light and energy, is passed on. Each time that human being comes into contact with another human being it spreads. It's like a positive virus. The energy of Star Magic is so potent, so powerful, it's desperate to expand. It flows up, out, in to the Star Magic Matrix, from each human being without human touch. Now it has started you cannot stop it. It will ebb and flow throughout each atom in the Universe and enlighten, heal and transform humanity. Star Magic is the most powerful transformational tool available, yet it cannot be held, touched or grasped. It's intangible yet "realer" than my fingers that are pressing the buttons on this keyboard right now, sharing these words with you.

This energy can't be read in words. It can only be felt, known, remembered and downloaded. You can use this book as a healing tool by reading it, or simply holding it in your hands. I strongly suggest that after every chapter or each new healing way you read and feel, that you stop for a moment and sit with the energy and the awareness that surrounds it. Contemplate it. Let the magic filter deep within you. Magic really does exist and miracles really do happen. Now you are going to experience it first-hand.

Star Magic is more than just a healing modality. It's a lifestyle. This is going to be an experience where you make up the rules of the game. We are going to, together, play the right-brain game of life and create new realities based on intuition and trust. You are going to remember the power of alchemy, and magic and miracles will be words associated with your presence.

I am just a kid from the streets. I am no different from anyone else on this planet. I have simply been on a journey and was not willing to stand down in the face of adversity. I carried on exploring, climbed mountains, learned to turn obstacles into opportunities, remembered how to decipher the truth and discovered my power. I am going to ensure you do the same.

Star Magic not only has the potential to heal people. It can and will heal the entire planet. My mission is to share this with the world and create an unstoppable wave of love that cradles and inspires the entire human race.

Are you ready to love? Are you ready to heal? Are you ready to remember?

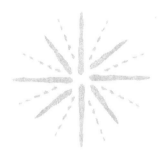

PART 1

1

Soul Technology

Star Magic is the most powerful technology available in this Universe. It's still in its infancy, and even now with the incredible ability I have remembered, there is still room for massive growth and technological advancements. I have seen some of them in my journeys, and it won't be long until I have remembered how to master these gifts and share them with you.

Star Magic is soul technology. It never breaks. It never crashes. It just expands, organically, getting better, becoming stronger and working faster with less effort. What's beautiful about the healing potential of Star Magic is that it has no detrimental effect on the environment or the human being that is being healed. No animals are needed to sacrifice to see how it will work. It is pure, it originated out of love – it is a gift from the creator of our Universe. God, Spirit, Infinite Intelligence, Source Energy, whichever label you decide to put on it.

Throughout this book I will refer to each of the above. When I do I am referring to energy or love. The power within the invisible. The space. It's the space after all that creates everything. It's the space between the notes that creates the music, the space between the bars that cages the lion and the space between the in and out breath that keeps you alive. There is enough energy within a cup of space to power the entire world – forever. So if there is that much power in a cup of space, imagine what you will be able to accomplish, once you harness the infinite power of Star Magic.

Star Magic has five mission-critical ingredients. I will share them with you now and will discuss them in detail later on.

1. **Love**
2. **Intention**
3. **Imagination**
4. **Knowing**
5. **Light**

These five ingredients, when used correctly, wisely and intelligently, carry the strength to create new worlds, new YOU-Niverses, and new galaxies. If Star Magic carries this much power, then healing yourself should be easy, and it will be. Open your mind, listen to your heart and feel the words and information that I share with you. Don't believe anything written on these pages – please, for your sake. Don't take anything on trust.

I would like you to experience what I share with you. Feel this information, go into it, deeply, and once it feels right, run with it. Try the Star Magic ways I share with you, experience them fully and know, deep within your heart and soul, that you are remembering the truth.

You are probably wondering how I discovered such a powerful gift? I am not going to go into my life story in this book. You can read about that in my books *Into the Light* or *The Vortex of Consciousness* (yet to be published). What I will do is say this. There was a time when I believed in Maya, in the illusion of the surface world. There was a day when I lived every waking second in a trance, driven by the material world of form. My ego was running the show, my mind was being controlled and I lived to make money, buy fast cars, build businesses and do it all thinking it would make me happy. I earned more money, built bigger businesses, travelled more and more, earning and spending and nothing ever made me happy.

Now, I want to make it very clear that you should experience this world of form fully. You should feel being human on every level, and remember, one very important factor as you do. It's just an experience. Everything is an experience. There is no good or bad. There just is. It is what it is and that is, it just is. The sooner you realize that you are energy or light as are all things, the happier you will be. There is no separation. We are one. United we stand. Divided we fall. Race, religion, colour, class OR language cannot separate energy or light. It simply gives the illusion of separation, exacerbated by the ego.

So how did I come from this material loving world, driven by my ego and discover the extraordinary power of Star Magic? It was a long road, a perilous journey. It started with a road accident and this I will share with you, as this day rocked and changed my world.

It was the early hours of the morning, between 4am and 5am. I was asleep in the passenger seat of an old Volkswagen taxi, travelling to Bucharest airport, in Romania, with my wife and our two children. It was the end of a two-week holiday, after visiting my wife Laura's family. All of a sudden I heard a loud crash and woke up, blurry eyed, full of adrenaline to see shattered glass flying, wind rushing against my face and the taxi swerving from side to side.

I remember thinking to myself *"boy we are in a serious accident"*. I was expecting the car to either hit the oncoming traffic or flip over, and then all of sudden, we came to a grinding halt. I looked around and Laura was sat there, with a mouth full of glass, holding onto our son Josh. My daughter Aalayah was underneath the driver's seat. They were all OK, apart from the shock. Then I turned to my left and saw the taxi driver, in shock, staring into space. I then turned and looked in front of me: there was a hole in the windscreen and my head was extremely sore. I didn't realize how sore, until the adrenaline had worn off shortly after.

Whenever the story comes up in conversation, even now, Aalayah my daughter says *"your head was bleeding wasn't it Dad?"*, but it wasn't. This is how she remembers it. If it wasn't my blood, then whose blood was it?

I opened the car door and got out. Time seemed to have come to a standstill, it felt eerie but calm. The country road we were on was empty; no cars were around, not one. I looked up the road about twenty to thirty metres, and saw two ladies on the floor. A little further up the road was what looked like another human being, a body lying there motionless. What had happened I asked myself? A million thoughts were flying through my head, and at the same time, my mind felt empty.

What had happened is this. Three ladies were crossing the road early in the morning on their way to work. Our taxi was going too fast, and there were no street lamps, on this old Romanian country road. The ladies stepped out to cross and our taxi came hurtling along, and hit the first lady clean on. She came through the windscreen, hit me in the head and then got sucked back out and flipped up over the car. The second lady's ankles got caught, and were in a terrible state, and the third lady was physically unharmed.

As I walked up the road, I walked past the two ladies that were to my left as there was really nothing I could do. A nearby factory worker was already on the scene, and had called the emergency services. I proceeded to walk up the road, towards the body lying on the floor. As I got near, I knew she was dead. I got within a few metres and saw her legs wrapped up over her head. She was in a real mess.

Daylight had just started to break through and the whole scene seemed so surreal. There were fields both sides of the road and nothing else bar an old factory, still in use. What was extraordinary about this event was what I saw before my eyes, as I approached the body. I saw the lady's soul, an etheric-like energy source, which was hovering above. I couldn't believe what I was seeing with my own eyes. I shook my head, and still the energy source remained there.

What was only seconds seemed like an eternity, as time stood still! It then vanished, fizzled out and went on its merry way, back into the vastness of the Cosmos. I was experiencing or witnessing, first-hand, what happens after death. I saw the total connection or dis-connection in this case, between the body and the soul. It hit me like a high-speed train, full blast.

I looked down at the body and looked up to the sky. I looked back down again at the body on the floor and said, thank you. I felt so privileged to have been a part of this and to see first-hand what happens after death, and to see the total separation. I realized there and then that the body is just a vessel, to carry the soul in this lifetime, and when the time comes for them to part, the soul moves on. No love is lost. It was like it (the soul) had taken an old car to the scrap heap. I had seen dead bodies before, but this was different. For the first time in my life I understood the truth.

This event, along with three others that happened in quick succession, was instrumental in taking me on my inward spiritual journey. They catapulted me onto a new and inspiring path, where I discovered my true purpose, my destiny, the reason I came to this planet, the truth about the world, and the vast complexity of the multi-dimensional YOU-Niverse, we live and play the game of life in.

This event led me on a journey and over the course of time, all the pieces of the Star Magic puzzle slotted into place. My mission now is to enhance the lives of one billion people. I will be setting up eleven Star Magic Facilities around the world – healing centres where people come to remember. I will take everyone through the same process that I went through, in the Ancient Mystery Schools of Egypt.

When you come to understand/know Star Magic you will be able to travel into the future, which is really the "now" in a different space. You will be able to see possible future scenarios and make decisions now, ones that will lead you and the human race to peace. Create peace internally now and peace will be created externally now. You are, after all, a co-creator of your own reality. (It's important that you know peace and never desire it. By desiring it you create the opposing cross-currents, distortions.)

By the very nature of desiring peace you create its opposite, non-peace or war. To create peace, you must know peace. The more one tries to create peace and eliminate war, the greater the distortion in our perception. By knowing peace and love, you know the truth and the less distorted you become. Once there is zero distortion within your own field, you will become whole and know your power.

This is how I know I will be creating thirteen Star Magic Healing Centres: in North America, South America, Moorea, Africa, the United Kingdom, New Zealand, Egypt, Canada, Portugal, France, Russia, Romania and at a location in Asia that has not been revealed as of yet. I have seen them all fully developed. It's incredible. This is the power that Star Magic gives you. I am still learning, or remembering, as I like to say. Once I have remembered a little more I will be setting up my first one, our first one.

You are going to gain clarity, confidence, and strength and more importantly you are going to love yourself on a deep level. The most important relationship you can have is the one with yourself, and Star Magic will ensure you truly develop this relationship, open your heart and love yourself, unconditionally.

You will release all blocks and open the door; you will create space and harness your creativity, which in turn will allow your full human potential to rise. You will be inspired. Inspired is "in spirit". Spirit within. It's this spirit within that will move you, guide you, and steer you in the direction to fulfil your destiny. As it does, enjoy every moment. Live fully. Be in the now and be enthusiastic. Enthusiasm is a great word, given to us by the Greeks. It translates as God within. It's this enthusiasm that inspires you. God within. In spirit. Words are far deeper than our logical human perception.

When you follow the ways in this book your world will open up. Your extraordinariness will surface, and when it does you will see life completely differently. You will see it as I do. I see no separation. I see no boundaries. I see no division. All I see is a vibrating mass of particles in continuous movement – one unified field. My world consists of geometry, infused together with love.

When you open your eyes and you see this too, you have journeyed deep enough, and are ready to experience the truth. The truth isn't always pleasant. To know that everything you have ever known is false, can be a hard pill to swallow. But to know that once the illusion drops away, an even greater source of intelligence will be revealed, one that offers you ultimate power, the power of alchemy, will fill your heart with joy.

You are a living breathing technology. Once you activate the dormant parts of your brain and ignite sleeping DNA with light codes, you will be this technology. You will be able to read Star Language, which is the language of light and sound. You will have access to the Universal Database where knowledge of all things past, present and future lies. You will be Soul Technology. Technology of the soul.

When the lady came through the windscreen and collided with me in the car that morning, I feel she activated an instant recognition. A recognition within myself that I am powerful, a deep knowing that enabled me to remember our natural and hereditary talents, gifts, ways. I became Soul Technology. I re-ignited elements of my own genetic make-up. I connected fully, once again with the stars. *Every atom in your body came from a star that exploded.* Maybe the atoms in your hands came from a different set of stars than the atoms in your legs? We wouldn't have been here if stars hadn't exploded because all of the elements – carbon, nitrogen, oxygen, iron, all things that matter for the evolution of life were not created at the beginning of time.

They were created in the loving nuclear furnaces of the stars and the only way for them to get into your body is if those stars were kind enough to explode. The stars exploded so you could be here.

You are Star Dust, my friend.

2

How Did My Healing Journey Begin?

Some people I speak to have known since they were young that they possessed certain extrasensory gifts. They were aware of beings in between worlds and they were fortunate enough to have parents that encouraged it – unlike the majority of parents that unknowingly tame their children's inner child.

Other healers or spiritual workers I know became aware of these gifts later on. I was very much the same. I didn't grow up thinking I want to be a healer. Some kids want to be a fireman, a doctor or a farmer. I wanted to be a rugby player but that was short lived. Not once though did I ever consider becoming an energy healer, let alone remembering and developing the most powerful energy healing modality in the world.

It started one day (shortly after the car crash in Romania) when my wife Laura, had a severe migraine. She was in bed. She couldn't move, let alone open her eyes because the pain was so intense. For some reason, I felt I could take it out. So I placed my hand on her head, and immediately, I saw the headache. The best way I can describe it is that I saw the energy of the head-ache, and attached my hand to it. It was green. I began to slowly lift my hand away from her head, and I saw the energy lifting. It rose up in sync with my hand and then just popped out of her head.

Laura jumped up off the bed and it was as though she never had a migraine in the first place. Laura described it like this, *"I felt Jerry put his hand on my head and then stuff was moving around. It was a bit like a misty cloud, moving up, and then over my head. I then felt him pull it out."*

Whether it is a migraine, a tumour or broken bones that are being healed/transformed I find it fascinating, hearing the descriptions of personal healing experiences, and how they perceived the healing. Later in the book I will share with you some interesting stories such as instantaneous tumour removals, fibromyalgia disappearing, facial reconstruction from serious road traffic accidents and much more.

After taking the headache from my wife's head, nothing much else happened for a few months. I was probably too busy being busy to stand still, create some space and feel the messages coming from the YOU-Niverse, to guide me on my healing journey. Then my family and I moved to New Zealand and soon after arriving, a friend of mine, back in the UK, was involved in a serious road traffic accident. She was taken to Frenchay Hospital in Bristol and was in intensive care. The doctors had told her partner that she may never walk again, and could be in hospital for at least a year.

I got a call from her partner asking if I could help. I thought to myself, how can I help? She's in the UK and I'm in New Zealand, how can I possibly help from here? Then my intuition took over. I felt that I should go and lie on the bed and get some of my crystals out. I lay the crystals across different chakras (energy points) on my body, and then, within a heartbeat, I was inside her hospital room and energy started pouring from my hands. It was as though I just knew what to do. I started mentally putting her body back together again.

I did this every day or every other day for a few weeks. My friend walked out of hospital in twelve weeks, with the use of a zimmer-frame, and within a few months, she was walking unaided. The doctors were amazed at her speedy recovery. It was a miracle in their eyes. At this point I didn't know whether I had actually done anything to help or not. I was still questioning and not trusting.

The most amazing part about this story was what she told me when she phoned me, soon after coming out of hospital: *"Jerry, I woke up one night and looked at the side of my bed and said, what are you doing here?"*

She was talking to me. She saw me with her physical eyes, exactly where I had imagined myself. Not a metre to the left or right, but exactly where I had been transported to. I thought to myself that there is more to this imagination stuff than meets the eye. Imagination is actually reality.

At the time I owned a health and fitness centre in New Zealand and was too busy being busy with that, to think about healing. I actually feel that the health and fitness centre was also a catalyst for me, wanting to help people, but I didn't realize this for a few more years. In actual fact I had started healing people then, in a different way to how I do now, but I was healing people none the less.

Shortly after this incident I was meditating in my friend Michael's copper pyramid, in his back garden. As I was meditating Jesus appeared in front of me. At the same time my feet turned to balls of fire and he said, *"Jerry, you*

can walk anywhere and be safe. Be fearless and go forth." I didn't know what
he meant. I was in the flow just observing. Then a set of steps appeared, or a
staircase, with a wooden door at the top. I walked up the steps and through
the door. I was sat in the Last Supper.

I was Matthew, one of Jesus's disciples, and Jesus was there, giving, what
I assumed was his last supper sermon. Then, in the background, through
a window, I saw a space ship. A gigantic spaceship hovering outside the
window. It was vivid. "More real" than real. No questions, at that moment,
I really was Matthew, looking out of the window, viewing the craft of one of
the extra-terrestrial space communities. After a period of time, I am not sure
how long, I popped back into my body, and was sat in the garden, inside this
copper pyramid.

Another event happened in this pyramid, which one might find a little
stranger, yet was magnificently real. I was meditating one day with my eyes
open. I was at peace, drifting through space and then all of a sudden, what
I would refer to as a space pod, landed next to the pyramid. A humanoid-
looking being, with intense but friendly energy asked me to get inside. So I
took my light and jumped inside the vehicle. We travelled at speeds I cannot
describe and landed on Alpha Centuria, one of my home planets from many
years ago.

As I stepped out from the aircraft my feet felt the ground and it was warm.
I needed a pair of shades as it was bright. There were many beings there to
welcome me, as though I had arrived home after a long holiday. I felt so at
home and at peace.

The technology on this planet was super-advanced. It was also very
clean. Zero pollution. I stayed for what seemed like hours and hours. I was
taken into some kind of structure and introduced to the chief. That is the
only way I can describe it. He/she, I am not sure, touched me on my head
and shoulders. It was like being knighted. This being said to me, *"You are
ready."* As my head was touched I received information. It was like a huge
bright, very light golden stream of information, flowed into my consciousness, through his touch. I was paralyzed as this information came down and
flooded into me. I could see codes, which made no sense whatsoever. It was
a combination of numbers, images and some sort of strange alphabet light
layered within the streams of light. I was receiving some sort of download.

Once this had taken place I was quickly escorted back (more like being
frog-marched) to the space pod. We jumped inside and within what seemed
like seconds, I was back in the garden, sat inside the pyramid.

It was after moving back to the UK, a year or so later, that my healing journey went into overdrive. I was out running one Sunday morning and I saw some fairies flying around a tree. I stopped to look at them. Then from nowhere an angel appeared. He told me his name was Archangel Gabriel and that I must adhere to my mission. A mission I chose as a light healer, before embarking on this journey, within this Earthly body. He told me to write a book, called *Into the Light*. So I ran home and opened my computer, and this book poured out. I would write every morning between five and seven a.m., as instructed.

It wasn't until I had finished the book that I realized why I had to write it. As I was downloading the information from the book, I was also downloading light, from this beautiful angel. The angel was acting as a facilitator to pass information to me. The experience on Alpha Centuria, and with Angel Gabriel, changed my frequency. I had been installed with information, light codes, which were to be used for healing.

Shortly after this event I was walking along one day and I saw some sort of hieroglyphics floating through the air. I also saw geometric signs (what I call Space-Geometry) and symbols (but different from any geometry I had seen in this human world) as clear as day, hovering and moving through the space. I would blink and then open my eyes again and the shapes would move. They would be there but in a different place. It was as though they had re-arranged themselves to create a new piece of information. The information I was viewing was the same as the codes I saw in the download on Alpha Centuria. Things started slotting into place.

These signs and symbols, in terms of my left brain, made no sense. I tried to analyze what was happening but it was useless. So I listened to my intuition, which told me to meditate deeply. So the next morning I woke early and spent two hours sat in my meditation room. After a few moments I was walking down a tunnel, through a set of corridors and across a stony floor, sprinkled with sand. I went through a set of doors and tunnels and more doors and then walked into a classroom. There were lots of people sat, at what I would describe as tables, looking at a man. He was like a teacher. He was unravelling a bunch of scrolls that were lying on a large flat surface.

As he was unravelling them and showing us (both my son Josh and I) the picture and symbols contained on each scroll, I came out of my meditation, and quickly scribbled them down and then wrote their meaning. This is where I got a part of the image for my Star Magic logo. This image, I was told by the teacher in this room, meant Healing Magic.

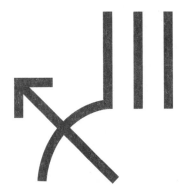

Star Magic symbol

The rest of the image came later (see also color insert).

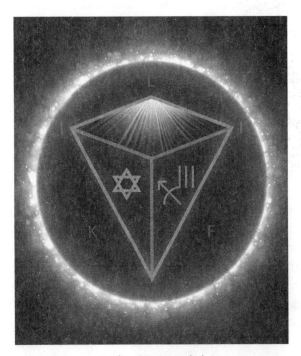

Healing Magic symbol

When I was shown these images, no one spoke, yet there was a clear and precise dialogue taking place. I was inside an Ancient Mystery School and was being taught (guided to remember) Star Magic. The magic part of the name comes from the healing magic symbol I was shown. The star part comes from space. I know, from being in these Ancient Mystery Schools, with one of the greatest teachers that has ever graced these mystical Earthly planes that each one of us, originally came from the stars. We are all extra-terrestrial beings that are here on this Earth plane for a short time, to learn about being human, to interact, to connect and to love in a world of chaos and mayhem – what I refer to as a jungle reality – caused by the illusory aspect of separation.

I spent months in these classrooms learning and my son Josh, used to come with me. He could see and feel just as clear as I could. It was a real pleasure to share these experiences with him. Together we discovered so much more about the pyramids' hidden secrets. If you're interested read my book *The Vortex of Consciousness*.

Soon after learning, journeying and remembering, people with diseases, discomfort, illness or injury just seemed to filter into my life. I felt compelled to help them. So I offered, as it was a chance to test out the information I had been remembering. Everything that I was trying was working. It was incredible. From there I decided to open up shop fully. I devoted all my time and energy to healing and it just happened. I was in alignment with my life destiny and so life aligned itself with me, and clients started to come.

Another important catalyst at this time, was again, Laura. She came home with a book from the library one day, read it and then said I should read it. It was about an Irish healer called Joe the Diviner. Now, with me finding my real mum at the age of twenty-five and knowing my ancestors were all Irish, this book really resonated with me. Joe had these abilities and had created a business from it, so why couldn't Jerry? Reading this book gave me an extra boost of confidence to set forth on this mission to heal the planet.

I quickly developed workshops, and now, I have an international client base, including people that I would never have expected. Now I expect nothing and extraordinary things effortlessly flow into my life. When you're in alignment life really does flow. And that is my mission, to assist as many human beings as possible on their inward journey to connect with source energy, the infinite intelligence that created you, me and everyone else on this planet. *Star Magic is the key*. It is so potent. It has helped thousands of people align spiritually and very quickly.

I also started to see angels. They would create a scaffolding-like structure around my body. It was made from light and connected me to what I refer to, as the Channelled Network of Light (CNL). This network connects you to the Universal Database and allows the flow of information to run into your consciousness, uninterrupted. Receiving these major downloads, spending months in Egyptian Mystery Schools and being connected to the CNL were all instrumental in me remembering these abilities that we are all capable of remembering.

> *When you are inspired by some great purpose, some extraordinary project, all your thoughts break their bonds, your mind transcends limitations, your consciousness expands in every direction and you find yourself in a new, great and wonderful world. Dormant forces, faculties and talents come alive, and you discover yourself to be a greater person by far than you ever dreamed yourself to be.*
>
> — PATANJALI

These words written by the Indian Mystic are so profound, so deep and authentic. When you journey within, connect with the spirit that created you and allow your uniqueness to rise to the surface, magical events, one after the other start to happen. A trail of synchronistic happenings – as if by the wave of a magician's wand – start to shape and mould your world.

Be inspired, my friend.

3

Five Magical Ingredients

When a baker bakes a cake they have to put specific ingredients in to allow the cake to form. Without those ingredients the cake won't taste right, or the texture will be wrong. No one actually cooks or bakes the cake once the ingredients are put into it. You simply put it in the oven and watch it rise, harden in texture, smell delicious and eventually this lovely cake is taken from the oven, allowed to cool and is ready to be eaten.

Bakers don't sit there wondering if the cake will turn out OK. Well, they may if it's their first few times but eventually they will "trust". They don't panic, thinking that it will be too soft, too hard or too sweet. They mix the ingredients together, never once thinking that there is more flour or sugar in one part of the bowl than the other. In the ingredients go, and then off to the oven with the mixture; to let nature take its course.

Star Magic works in very much the same way. There is a set of specific ingredients. You mix those ingredients together and then the light and energy goes to work and heals the human being in question. You, me, or whoever is doing the healing is simply facilitating the process. It's the energy, source intelligence or consciousness that does the work. Light of an extra-terrestrial nature is the tool. The five mission-critical ingredients that make the Star Magic cake are:

1. **Love**
2. **Intention**
3. **Imagination**
4. **Knowing**
5. **Light**

1. Love

Love is the most powerful, measurable force in the YOU-Niverse. It's an energy. An energy so powerful that it can alleviate the painful conditioning from any human being, and ignite their inner healing spark. After all, we all have the ability to self-heal. We were designed that way. Love is the most powerful healer. Love has the courage and the strength to journey deep within our cells and then even deeper into our soul, to bring us face to face with our greatest fears.

By facing these fears and allowing old emotional patterning to surface, we can observe these emotions, sit with them and then let them go. Love has the power to create the perfect environment whereby profound healing can take place.

There are a number of ways, basic and advanced, that you can utilize to allow pure unconditional love to filter through, and be the driving force behind every healing session, whether it be for you or on a client that you are facilitating the healing of and I will be showing you all of these ways later in the book. Love is like invisible glue. It lies in every atom, in every cell of the body; it permeates all matter and vibrates throughout all space. Love is energy and energy is love. Love is the essence that bonds the ingredients of Star Magic, the same way in which it bonds worlds, YOU-Niverses and galaxies together. Dropping into your heart space is the only way to activate the facilitation of prominent healing.

2. Intention

Nothing in this world happens without intention. I can't put one foot in front of the other without intention. I can have all the ability in the world but unless I engage that ability, nothing will happen. You could have the fastest formula one racing car in the world and the best driver, but unless that driver puts his intention into driving the car fast, holding it in the bends and manoeuvring around his opponents, he hasn't got a hope in heaven of winning the race.

My intention when I am about to facilitate a healing is extraordinary. I communicate with the energy and the light through my intention and direct it in the direction of the human being that needs healing. I also use my intention to summon the help of spirit guides, the ones whom will be best suited to the particular healing in front of me. I also have an open intention. It's never focused on one particular thing. I will say to the YOU-Niverse, *"Please show me what I don't know to help me facilitate the healing of this incredible human being."* By asking for what I don't know I open myself up to the sea of infinite possibilities.

Consciousness is intelligent. So the energy, my spirit guides, they know what needs to be done and will bring forth the best surgeons or beings for the job. Use your intention wisely. It can create chaos and mayhem just as easily as it can create health, healing and a kind and blissful reality. When using your intention always ensure it is for the greatest good and not specific.

If you ask for something specific, it will happen but what about everything else outside of that? Be open and allow for anything to happen. Don't limit the sea of infinite change, the realm of infinite possibilities. Be like a child when facilitating healing and play. Drop into the healing zone (something we will discuss later on) and co-create the new reality with light (information) as you go.

3. Imagination

Imagination is real. Don't ever forget that. What is in your mind is your reality, in another space. And remember there is no such thing as time or distance, so everything is now. Past, present and future are one, all happening simultaneously in the now. If a client comes to me with a tumour (after being presented with scan results or the news from the doctors) and I look inside their stomach and see no tumour, which one of us is right? We both are. We are simply looking through different perspectives. There are a multiple number of possible future outcomes that are governed by the choices we make.

Healing is no different. I can choose to manipulate reality and remove a tumour from someone's body. I can use my imagination to create an environment, where the healing takes place or an operation is performed. When it comes to healing it works in a myriad of ways – this is what I love about working with energy and light. I could remove a tumour from a client and in an instant the emotional cause behind the tumour releases too. In another reality, it's simply not there. We can flip between realities instantaneously. Our power is in the knowing.

In other situations, a dis-ease may be removed and over the course of the next days, weeks, possibly months, the emotional baggage that caused the dis-ease, in the first place, rises to the surface and the human being in question will have to sit and observe those emotions and let them pass. This isn't always easy, however, it's often part of the deal.

What's interesting for me, as 90% of my healing is done at a distance, is the use of imagination in terms of body positioning. If I am in the UK and you are in California or Russia, I can sit in one position and work on your feet. I can then flip your entire body around and work on your head in a heartbeat, because wherever I put my focus is where the energy and light will go.

I can also bi-locate to your home or wherever you are and work on you. I can bi-locate and sit by your feet, your chest and your head and do it very quickly. Quite often I will bi-locate to your place of healing and pick your body up with the help of a dragon I work with. Together we will transport your body to Egypt. I will discuss this in depth later on as it's a huge part of my work.

I can also allow other multi-dimensional versions of me to help with the healing. So I can break off into different forms. It's like having three, four or five Jerrys working on you at once. I love the magnitude of this work – I'm consistently co-creating new realities.

4. Knowing

Knowing is imperative. You have to know that what you are doing is working. Or has already worked. Don't set goals when you are healing with Star Magic – know that the energy and light is working, create your intention, infuse it with love, know it's working, use your imagination and then let the light go to work and do what is necessary.

Knowing is also feeling, and when you're creating with Star Magic, you must still your mind, come into your heart and feel everything. Feel and see the insights, feel and see the visions, and know that what you are sensing is direct knowledge from the Universal Database. Whatever you see and feel may not make any sense rationally, logically; the ego will try and screen it out.

So you must know, be still and aware and feel the vibrations floating into your consciousness, brought to you through Star Language. Star Language is the ability to read the information contained in light and sound frequencies. It's the ability to decipher the truth amongst the illusion. The more you practise the better you become, the higher your level of understanding, and with greater accuracy you will be able to interpret the ancient art of geometric codes.

This world is made of codes. Our brain is a biological computer. When you master Star Magic (by becoming it) you will be able to change the software programmes in another human being's biological computer in seconds, installing a new and empowering programme that creates health, confidence, clarity, abundance, acceptance and much more. I have a set of codes or frequencies for everything. I remembered them in the Ancient Mystery Schools of Egypt. I will be sharing some of them with you, when you get to the chapter titled The Secret Recipe.

Stop believing. Start knowing.

Knowing is also not knowing. What do I mean? Well, you know that Star Magic will work but you don't necessarily know how. And let me tell you this. It's perfect when you don't know. I always get questions and a lot of the time, my answer is, *"I don't know."* Does it affect my ability to heal? No! Can you see electricity? No! Do you buy it? Yes! Learn to be comfortable with not knowing what and why you know. Feel it, experience it but don't try and rationalize it. Love and play with it, dance and run with it.

Remember this: as soon as you think you know, you limit yourself – you must know that it is a given, that the outcome, which is for the greatest growth of the human being/client in question, is a given, but also know that you don't know what that outcome is. By giving yourself this freedom of movement you open the gateway to the sea of infinite possibilities. This is where miracles happen.

If someone I am facilitating the healing of asks for a specific outcome, it very well may happen. Is that best for them? Who knows! And they will never know either because they have confined the explosion of beauty and the informative codes contained within the light, to access their being at one level, and manipulate their light codes to marry up with a specific outcome. Anything outside of this has been left in a different reality. A reality that the client was not open to. The best healing sessions I have facilitated are the ones that have no specific outcome in mind. Be free and leave room to explore.

5. Light

One thing that is important to point out at this stage is that Star Magic is not about running energy though your body. It's about utilizing light. Light is a source of energy, of course, but we are working in the realm of imagination and intuition, not the running of energy through our bodies and into our clients.

Light is not just light. Light is the source of all knowledge. Love and light go hand in hand. Love is creation, the creative force, the glue, the power. Light is information. Love without light does not work. Light without love does nothing. Love, the creative force takes light, the information and works its magic with it.

Love takes the information contained within the light and infuses it deep into the cells of the human being (at a level of light) that is being healed. We are, after all constructed from light, geometry, shapes and symbols. Our physical human bodies are an illusion. This light then travels deep into the cells; it connects with the spiritual intelligence and starts to change the DNA structure with the human being that is being healed.

This is the extraordinary power of Star Magic. It goes to the root cause of the issue. Not the block caused by a certain trauma in this lifetime. That is just surface level, box standard healing. Star Magic goes way beyond. Star Magic enables the light to go so deep into the cells/atoms that it shifts the genetic conditioning from thousands, if not millions of years ago.

The light, when used in Star Magic goes way back to the start, wherever that may be. Years and years of genetic conditioning is brought to the surface. It either passes away quickly or the human being in question has to sit with the emotions, observe and learn to let them go. Star Magic uses the light to bypass everything logical. Any mind-made barriers are no match for the light frequencies in Star Magic.

If you pull a weed up from the garden it will grow back again. Why? Because you left the root in the ground. It's why cancer patients often have their tumours cut out and then they return. Why? Because you can't cut the emotions out. To do that you must go deep, and this is where the space codes within the light offered through Star Magic, come into play. Light is an integral piece of the Star Magic puzzle. Light contains all possibilities.

Energy healing should actually be called light healing or a more accurate way of describing it would be information exchange. Really and truthfully that is all that is happening. Light is information and the frequencies that I bring forth are light frequencies. It's not energy as such. I am not running energy when I am facilitating the healing of another human being. I am using light to communicate. I am facilitating the exchange of information. This in turn creates healing.

Mix these five mission-critical ingredients together and you carry within your healing tapestry, an un-wavering power. The power to create miracles, now and forever more. Within your life and the lives of others. Every one of us can create with Star Magic. Mixing these five ingredients together and then letting go will create a pathway for you to explore the YOU-Niversal toolbox. You can step outside of the box and be free to surf the intelligent sound and light codes that make up our world.

A lady contacted me about her sister's scans from her doctor showing an eroding oesophagus, which, from what I read in the report, was an infection in the pipe connecting the mouth to the stomach. This lady was in hospital and dying slowly. Her oesophagus was black and closed and had been for some time. In every healing session I always ask to be shown what I don't know and then let go. I am then shown different realities that I help co-create. In this particular incident one of my guides showed me a green frog. This frog then spat some venom into a jar. A blue light then came down from space and into the jar and mixed with the frog's venom. I then took out a syringe and sucked the mixture up. I injected it into the lady's neck, at the back in the centre. It felt like the best place to inject it. All of this took about ten minutes.

The next day I received an e-mail letting me know that she was no longer in pain and had stopped vomiting. Her throat was clear and she had started eating for the first time in weeks. The doctors were bemused. Now, in my eyes I did nothing. The family was asking me what I did. The doctors wanted to know how she had gotten better. It was unexplainable in their eyes.

I would have loved to have seen the look on the doctor's face when I said I mixed imaginary frogs' venom with a blue light from space and then injected it into the back of her neck. Ha ha! But that is what happened. When you drop into your heart and play with what comes into your consciousness and surrender to the illogical, miracles really do happen.

Star Magic will help you step outside of the proverbial box and use the tools you are not aware of, the ones that make a real difference. A difference you know nothing of.

4

Why Do People Get Ill?

People don't get ill. People do illness. You are a spiritual being created by love. Love knows no illness. You are a vibrating mass of particles. You are energy. You are light. Energy is continuously moving through form, into form, out of form and back again. Energy is expansive and is always on the move. If you look at me today I look like Jerry Sargeant. If you look at me next week I will look like Jerry Sargeant. In three weeks or a year's time, I will still look like Jerry Sargeant. All you are looking at is a pattern.

We are all patterns. What do I mean? Because we are energy and because energy is always on the move, it means that the energy inside of us is changing. I am new atoms, molecules, carbons and a variety of different chemicals, which are constantly changing. It's like a whirlpool in a stream. The whirlpool is always there but the water that is running through it is different. It's consistently different and not once does the same drop of water pass through the whirlpool.

If our bodies are always changing, being refreshed and rejuvenated by new energy, how is it possible for illness or dis-ease to hang around? It's actually impossible. Impossible that is in a body, with a mind thinking empowering thoughts. When our body does a dis-ease, it's simply that negative thoughts have bypassed our security system.

Our body is a highly advanced communication device that lets us know when something has slipped past our radar system, and caused unhappy or negative emotions, such as anger, hurt, jealousy, rejection and so forth. When we have negative thoughts, they generally lead to (if not vented, expressed and released) negative emotions because the mind and body are intrinsically linked.

You can harness these negative thoughts by living life in your heart, as an observer, watching yourself living in this life, instead of being caught up in the constant stream of illusory information. When you remember to observe your own mind, you can catch these thoughts in the process. You can clearly see them and so re-direct your thoughts and focus on to that which will empower you. Wherever your focus goes your energy surely follows.

Mother Teresa once said, "Please don't invite me to an anti-war demonstration." She knew that by going to an anti-war demonstration, even though it's anti-war, she would still be giving her focus to war, and so her energy would create more of it. It's actually important to create peace but to create peace you cannot want peace. As soon as you want it, by the very nature of wanting, you create separation and so, by default, you create its polar opposite, war or non-peace. To create peace, you must know and be peace.

I often get cases of women with breast cancer that work in breast cancer charities. They were perfectly healthy when they started work there, and because their entire focus has been on breast cancer, they manifest it themselves. They have created it with their thoughts. A constant stream of thinking about breast cancer. I knew a lady once, before I started healing, who had cancer and had her womb removed. Every week she would go to a ladies' cancer group and all they would talk about was the dis-ease. She got it back again and had a breast removed. Then she went back to the group again and again, it re-ignited and the other breast was removed. She wouldn't listen to her family's advice, and stop going to this weekly group. I am sure spiritually she is learning lessons and it's her journey. It's not for me to judge. It's her path. Acceptance of everyone, always, is important.

Learn to remember or re-direct your thoughts and you will control your emotions. If you have not yet mastered this or have a family member, friend or client that has a dis-ease due to these un-observed thought patterns then you must utilize Star Magic. We are conditioned from a very young age, by our environment, and this affects our behaviours, thought patterns and the way we see the world. I was fostered and eventually adopted as a child so rejection and a lack of love for self has been a huge challenge for me.

Especially when it came to following my true purpose in life – writing books, speaking publicly etc. Having to face my massive rejection issues. That, my friend, is the way the game was designed. To follow my heart and discover my destiny I had to face my greatest fear – and your most extraordinary version of yourself, always lives on the other side of your fears.

Also, our ancestors affect the way in which we think. Genetic conditioning is ingrained within our DNA, at a cellular level. Our bones also carry lifetimes of "stuff". If your mother was fearful of losing her husband, it's possible that you will be too. And it's possible that your grandmother and great grandmother all thought the same thoughts and had the same feelings, created by the same experiences. It's passed on down the line. Star Magic will give you the chance to break this chain, enable you to be free and offer freedom to your children, and your children's children.

Every dis-ease has an emotional cause. The majority of the time it's fear based or a lack of love based. Let me give you some examples. If someone has something simple such as stiffness in their body, it's usually due to their being rigid in their thinking. In other words, stiff thinking. If someone has something more severe such as cancer, it's usually because of deep-seated grief or the lack of love one has for the self – constantly eating away at oneself.

In the end the cancer eats the body away. It's just mirroring your internal way of viewing yourself. You are "doing" the dis-ease based on your thought processes. Spots are often an outburst of anger. Haemorrhoids, which is something I tend to deal with a lot, in men especially, are caused by anger at the past, not wanting to let go of what happened and in the end they feel overwhelmed with burden.

Every dis-ease has an emotional link. It's not actually necessary to know them all. It's not necessary to know any. You see, Star Magic bypasses everything logical, and goes to work and alleviates the so-called problem, at the deepest core level. The reason I am sharing this with you, is to help you understand, that because every dis-ease has an emotional link, it's simple to remove it. Move or change or shift the emotions and the dis-ease will dissolve. This can all be done at a level of light. Nothing logical is needed when one is creating using Star Magic.

What happens when sunlight shines on a shadow? The shadow disappears. That is all that is happening during healing. Star Magic journeys deep into the cells, and the soul of the individual, and goes fishing. It casts its rod into the archives of the Universal Database and catches the emotional cause that is causing harm. It reels it in and brings it to the surface, where the human being must observe it, and then let it go. In other words, shine light upon it. Sounds easy, right? Well it is. It's so easy. No need for long-winded treatments, and a concoction of pharmaceutical drugs, administered by the drug industry. Simply use Star Magic and transmute the root cause of the problem.

There are times when operations are necessary. In serious road traffic accidents for example. I have dealt with many of these. In a road traffic accident someone may be losing a lot of blood and may need a transfusion, and to be sown up. The bleeding will need to be stopped. In this case it's imperative for surgery, and a caring team of specialized doctors and nurses. You will see later on when I share some stories of people I have worked with, why doctors should bring in a Star Magic Facilitator to speed up the recovery process.

When the medical industry fully accepts Star Magic (which it will have to) healing human beings will be easier than easy. Teamwork is the key.

This is why we can all self-heal. Because the root cause of every dis-ease is held within us. Star Magic is direct, fast, and efficient and will hunt down that root cause, and give you, and everyone else on this planet, the chance to not only recover, but remove all blocks from within, so you can and will, truly flourish. Sometimes the blocks are resting in another reality or dimension.

If that is the case the block is accessed in exactly the same way, through light. Star Magic is an exploratory and fun process. You will remember how to play with it and track the root cause to whichever dimension or reality it may be hiding.

It will enable you to create/fulfil your own destiny, as your own prophecy attracting the business, the relationships, the health and wealth that you deserve. Whatever it is that your heart is drawn towards, Star Magic is the answer. Star Magic will create freedom on this planet for everyone.

One thing is certain. A pure connection with source/love = zero illness/dis-ease/problems of any kind.

5

The Universal Database

The energy source that drifted from the body after the accident (I shared with you earlier) was part of the great intelligence that created this YOU-Niverse. An intelligence so powerful, wise and whole. An intelligence that knows only love, compassion and purity. This living intelligence has manifested itself into many different forms, and is living life through all that you can see, and all that the naked eye cannot.

The YOU-Niversal intelligence created you, me, the stars, the moon, the sun, trees, animals, plants, fish, the rocks, flowers and birds and everything that is in between, the space. The space is the You-Niversal intelligence itself, and so are you. You are truly powerful. Extraordinary, in fact.

This energy source, the Universe, God, spirit, whichever label you decide to give to it is timeless, endless. It has no start, middle or end. It is no-thing and everything at the same time, and most importantly of all it is love, the most powerful, measurable force known to man. Jesus said God is love. I say Love is God. As humanity has travelled through the discrepancies of time, the awareness of our natural abilities to connect with source energy has faded, into not much more than obsolete.

The great intelligence has an infinite labyrinth of knowledge and wisdom, stored away in the invisible, in the non-material world. It's a large Universal Database available to each and every human being that graces this planet. Many old and wise beings of light that graced this planet, thousands of years ago, knew about this intelligence and were able to access it, just like you access a file on the hard drive of your computer. Men and women today, still have the capability, but the ability to access this knowledge is cloaked in layers of toxicity brought about by centuries of conditioning, indoctrination and unquantifiable manipulation.

Over many years, the mind, the most powerful computer there is, has been slowly laid to rest and people now only use approximately 10% of the human brain, much less in most cases. The Egyptians were a consciously aware race and knew the truth. They had access to and utilized the Universal Data base to live extraordinary lives. They didn't need telephones, cars, aircraft, computers, I-pads and all the other so called technological luxuries of this modern age. They could think a place and go there in their mind, and see what is happening. They travelled in Space-Ships and Mer-Ka-Ba's (a part of our human light body; we will discuss these later). They didn't need to open their mouths to communicate. They used Star Language and Star Magic.

The information lies deep within our DNA structure, waiting for our conscious awareness to heighten, much like carbon lying in the mountain, under extreme pressure, waiting to form diamonds and be discovered in the Earth by man. Diamonds have a price. Star Magic is priceless.

Way back when man was in touch or at one with his or her environment, they knew that the natural world could provide for them all that they needed to flourish. The world knew no pollution. Mother Earth was healthy and vibrant. The gifts that God bestowed on this planet were appreciated, respected and looked after. In this modern world we live in, there are a number of factors as to why we have forgotten our natural and hereditary power, given to us at birth by the great intelligence. The God particle that is in every man or woman, a part of our genetic make-up, is totally natural and is who we are at the core, a soulful energy source. A powerful soul connected to the totality of all life. Every particle contains all the information that has ever been and ever will be. These particles are within us all.

So why has this connection been lost? Why do most of us feel separate from our environment, like strangers in an alien land? Why do we struggle to be at one with our environment when we are just as much a part of the environment as the trees, plants and rocks?

For centuries the human race has been conditioned, instilled with fear and manipulated through a variety of external sources. You could call them the forces of darkness or maybe the forces embodied with a lack of light.

People with dark clouds surrounding the bright burning sunlight within them, controlled by their ego, who live to rule with power and control, thinking only of themselves and mentally enslaving the masses, by turning their attention towards a material, illusory world, that distracts the human race, from what is real and true - what is authentic and lies within each human being on this beautiful big blue planet, hovering in space.

Remember this. The only authority anyone has over you is the authority you give to them.

For centuries people have tried to teach with words. Yet still the human race pushes forward, headed for a global disaster. Or death by thinking. How about feeling? Feeling the love in your heart and by encompassing every thought with a projected image of oneness and cradled by the feeling of love. This will enable the human race to feel every word and thought and understand it authentically.

Some of our ancestors, for millennia, have carried waves of wisdom and the light of their own soul has been left as a legacy. Yet as a race we are so focused on the illusory material world that we have forgotten our ancient powers, perfectly orchestrated by Jesus, Buddha and many others.

The truth, a deep Knowing, will be brought about when one fulfils his or her own prophecy. It will only happen when one's life and relationship with the environment are expressed through faith, knowing, love and purpose. When one connects with nature, the life of that man or woman will be authentic and consciousness will flow through them. Every human being will be a vortex for consciousness. It will alter your perception and enable you to see the underlying truth, that you are powerful beyond measure. Star Magic will flow through your veins.

The technological world is structured in such a way that man keeps on inventing all sorts of mechanical devices and social orders, supposedly to make life easier. But in fact, any saving of labour is an illusion. Human beings are becoming robots of the technological world and Soul Technology has been forgotten. One rarely has the time to contemplate the essence of being or to listen to what another human being is saying, and has no time to reflect on his or her own destiny. We are literally breeding programmed robots that exist and have no desire to truly live. Star Magic is natural, and Soul Technology is nature, manifested into human form.

A flower does not exist, it lives. It comes into full blossom in spring and flourishes through the summer months, and its colours explode and fill the air with joy. This is how people should be. Exploding with joy and radiating love, exploding with excitement every day. After all we are just as natural as a flower. We are God's highest creation. Man has been blessed with a brain, a biological computer more powerful than any man-made device on this planet. It's time we regained our power, unlocked our true human potential and restored the world and Mother Nature to her former glory.

The YOU-Niverse communicates with you through vibration and rhythm, and so connecting with the Universal Database is established through feeling. By living in a state of conscious awareness, living with Wu Wei, in spontaneous flow. By living in the present moment and truly listening with your heart, you can connect to life once more, and be guided by nature. You can live within the flow of life and live happily ever after. After all, happiness is your birthright. It's your natural way of being. As you open, and allow Star Magic consciousness to flow, you will embrace the specialness and beauty of this vibrant and passionate world, once more. These extra-terrestrial light frequencies are full of resonating harmony.

The major contributor to all noble deeds is through human aspiration, and as you learn, develop and grow, by tuning into the vibration and rhythm of life, you will access this labyrinth of knowledge and wisdom, and your life purpose will become clear. Your outer world will change as you start to live an authentic life of love, compassion and the will to be open and connect. The magic that is, will flow through your life.

In humans thoughts are a part of our genetic memory. These thoughts have been turned to an acidic frequency over time. As soon as a human being becomes aware it's very easy to see which thoughts are our own, and which are the manipulative ones, sent to influence destructive behaviour.

To access your power and release your full human potential, it's imperative that you journey in, become aware and see the mist obscuring your vision. Then and only then will you harness Star Magic and Star Language.

Rumi once said the only thing that is real is that which doesn't change. When I look at me in the mirror now and compare it to photographs twenty years ago I look very different, but inside I feel the same. I don't feel any older. The only permanent part of this world is your spirit.

Last year my father passed over. I was there and carried him into bed not long before. He died in my arms. My mother and my sister were there too. Once he had transitioned, we called the funeral director. They came and took his body away. I helped them carry his body onto a trolley to be wheeled out to the waiting van. His body didn't feel any lighter; it was the same weight. Scientists have measured the weight of a body before death, and directly after, and there is no change in weight, yet the life force is gone. The spirit is timeless, endless, weightless. It cannot be measured. It's the immeasurable breathtaking beauty of love.

Everything you know, I know, and vice versa. Everything Jesus or Lao Tzu ever knew, so do you. We all know everything. We have simply forgotten how to tap into these resources. The resources and possibilities that are available to you, right now, are way beyond what most people can possibly fathom. The simple fact that our Universe is electromagnetic blows most people's minds.

Star Magic will give you the key to open this door of freedom, and be in the space of infinite possibilities.

In this space you will remember the power of bi-location, telepathic communication, distance healing, alchemy and so much more. Hold onto your seatbelt and get ready for the ride.

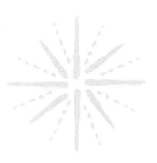

PART 2

6

A Learning Curve –
It's Not Always What You Think

I had a huge learning/remembering experience with a client of mine. In fact, each time I create with a client or a group I learn/remember, but this experience really hit home. In facilitating the healing of this client, I remembered so much, I feel I must share this – especially for all you healers reading this.

When someone comes to me with a particular dis-ease or ailment, that they want to eliminate, my first feeling is to cure them – to relieve them of all pain. That is what's right. That is what's meant to be. That isn't always the case however. Sometimes the healing that takes place, within a certain human being, is not exactly the way you perceive it to be. Let me explain what I mean by this.

It wasn't too long into the New Year and a dear friend of mine phoned me, and said a friend of hers, Rachel, had cancer. It was in her stomach, liver, spleen and was spreading. She had been diagnosed a long time previous, and it was getting more severe. She was laid up in bed and struggling to function, yet remained as cheerful as she could. She really inspired me to the depths of my soul, and beyond.

I first spoke with Rachel on a Sunday evening. We talked for some time. I asked her some questions about her life and she answered. It was clear to me, after feeling Rachel's energy for a few moments, that she had never loved herself. As she continued to describe her life it became even clearer.

We commenced the first healing that evening and did two more, one on the Monday morning and one on Monday evening. I wouldn't normally do this in quick succession, but Rachel's cancer was severe. We spoke briefly before each session, and after, I let her rest. When I phoned Rachel on the Tuesday morning she burst into tears. She said, "*Jerry, I actually love myself. For the first time in my life I truly love myself.*" She was so happy. These were tears of joy. It was an inspirational conversation. I could feel her heart beaming, overflowing with love.

We did another healing session that morning, and then spoke again on the Tuesday evening, before the next healing session. Rachel explained that her current divorce was really weighing her down and that she would like me to cut the emotional (energetic) cords, between her and her husband. We had discussed this energetic connection the previous day. I agreed, and a few minutes later we put the phone down, and I commenced the distance healing session.

I was working away and could see the cord right in the middle of her chest. It was very big, the size of her sternum. I started to remove it (we will discuss how to locate and remove energy cords later on). It was very thick, and took me around twenty minutes to get the entire cord out of her body and the emotional debris that came with it.

It left a gaping hole in her body. I had never taken an energy cord out that big before. It was a like taking a large oak tree from the ground, along with all of its roots. Imagine the size of the hole it would leave in the Earth.

Once the cord was out, I started filling the hole back up with light, or rather observing the light structures or patterns of light re-arrange themselves, and communicating with my guides at the same time.

I asked, *"What else do I need to do?"*

"Nothing", was the answer.

"Nothing?" I questioned.

"Yes", was the answer.

So in my mind I thought to myself, she is healed. *"Brilliant, the cancer will now move on as the emotions have been dealt with. She will make a full recovery and live happily ever after"*, was the conversation I had with myself at the time.

After the healing Rachel contacted my friend, the one who had introduced us. In her text message she wrote, *"a million thanks for Jerry. He has touched so many hearts and souls this week"*. Rachel then fell asleep and died. I was shocked when I got a message a few hours later. *"How could she be dead? You told me there was nothing more I had to do"* – as I looked up towards the heavens.

In the early hours of the following morning, I was meditating. As soon as I sat down Rachel came into my room. She said to me, *"Jerry, thank you so much. You helped me love myself for the first time in my life. You also cut the bonds that were stopping me moving back to spirit. I couldn't have stayed there on Earth. I have greater tasks to accomplish here in this space."*

She smiled at me and then left. Since that day Rachel has helped me with many a healing. As I am preparing myself, and calling upon the flow of Star Magic and the Star Team (something we will discuss later on), she drifts into my space, and helps me do what is necessary.

I am so grateful for her help and more importantly I am absolutely and totally overwhelmed by the lesson she taught me, in terms of healing, and your expectation towards it, along with an emotional attachment to any and every outcome.

The healing with Rachel was foreign to me in the sense that I felt being healed meant living/remaining alive. I then coined this phrase:

"Everyone can be healed but not everyone is ready. Everyone can be healed but not everyone can live."

The "not ready" part comes from secondary gain (which is when a human being gets benefits from being ill, such as sympathy and attention) and other various reasons why someone may not be ready to deal with their stuff. When you go to facilitate a healing, simply put the intention out there and then let the light and energy do the rest. Remember it is intelligent and knows what is for the greatest growth of everyone involved. Also, it's important that the receiver of the healing wants it. I often get phone calls where someone will say, *"Jerry, will you send my mum or my dad or my brother some healing?"* My answer is no. If they want some healing, they will call.

If someone is incapable of contacting me, due to their so-called condition, I will ask their inner self. (I prefer to use this term, inner self than higher self, as nothing is higher than you or me or anyone else. Higher self is a distraction, pointing humans in an external direction. All is within.) The same with babies and children. I will always ask. If it's a no, then I don't facilitate the healing. I don't always know why the answer is no, but I trust in my awareness and the intelligence that created us all.

Sometimes people will contact me themselves and I get a very strong, heavy feeling come over me, and I feel that I shouldn't do the healing. If that is the case then I leave it and have to say I am sorry but this healing isn't for your, or my greatest growth. This world, in terms of rational and logical, doesn't always make sense, especially when it comes to healing. If you want rational or logical go and be a mathematician or an English teacher.

A friend of mine's son was in hospital one day and the mother was beside herself. She phoned me up as I was walking into the gym and asked if I would do a healing. I said I will ask your son's inner self. So I did. I had just put my boxing gloves on and started hitting the bag and this young lad came into my space and said with so much force, *"no Jerry, my mum has to learn her lesson"* and then he disappeared. I jumped when he moved into my space like that. He was clearly ill to teach his mum and knew that my interference would be detrimental to her spiritual growth.

Star Magic is everything but logical. It's rooted in love. And we are all aware of the crazy things loves makes you do. Expect the unexpected.

In a situation like this it can be very easy for the ego to interfere. It may say things to you such as "but how can you leave this little boy in hospital" or "come on, Jerry, help him, for goodness sake". It will play on your heart strings. It can be very easy to interfere and help out, especially when children are concerned. We are talking beyond anything physical here, however. We never know what is for another human being's greatest growth.

Also, non-interference is the key to mastery. Being able to let everything around you unfold in the now, on its own as you observe is a real test of character. If you're a parent with children you will know exactly what I mean. Children should be allowed to bloom like flowers with zero interference.

7

Psychic Surgery

I had a call one Boxing Day from a gentleman named Mark. He had been in hospital for the last forty-eight hours fighting for his life. His blood tests showed E-coli and Peritonitis. Scans showed three Cysts in his intestine and a large growth.

The doctors told him if he made it through the next forty-eight hours, they would refer him to a surgeon, to have ten feet of his large intestine removed, and that he would have to have a bag fitted, for the rest of his life, to go to the toilet.

Mark did make it through the next forty-eight hours, contacted me, and explained the situation. I asked him to lie on the bed and relax. I centred myself in my meditation/healing space and I then went to work and entered Mark's room. He was in Coventry and I was in Cheltenham, England, more than fifty miles away. In my line of work, distance is irrelevant. I gave Mark a healing on this particular day and then another a week later.

Here is the story in Mark's words:

> Jerry asked me to lie on the bed and relax. I did so and then the room went ice cold. I saw two big shafts of light by the side of my bed and then it felt as though my body was being stretched out. I started to wonder what was happening and then from nowhere a Unicorn came and kissed me on my nose. It told me I would be OK. It didn't seem strange seeing a Unicorn, it felt right.
>
> I then found myself drifting and then looked up and I was in a room full of people. They looked like surgeons and they were all standing around looking at me. The building was tall, made of stone and ancient looking. It was Egypt. I felt my stomach being worked on and then a hand – it was Jerry's hand, up to the ends of his fingers – entered my stomach right where the major pain was. I am not sure how long this went on for as time just stood still. It could have been hours or minutes.

I then came around in my room and felt disorientated. I stood up, went to the bathroom and looked down at my stomach. There was a big scar across it. I couldn't believe it. I took a photo to show Jerry and my mum as it shocked me.

The second healing was very similar. I felt work being done on my stomach and also my spine as I had some major problems since falling in a horse race (ex-jockey) and being trampled on by several horses. I hadn't told Jerry about my back but he seemed to work on it anyway.

I went to the doctor in January and he almost fell off of his chair. He was amazed. The swelling in my stomach had gone and I was eating. No more diarrhoea and zero pain. He said I looked twenty years younger. Everyone was telling me I looked younger. I was due to see the surgeon on the 22nd February. My doctor said you don't need the operation anymore. I have had no more pain, no more tablets, my digestion is perfect. The lumps in my intestine have disappeared. My blood tests came back with no E-coli or Peritonitis. I was cured. It was a miracle.

People would refer to this as psychic surgery. For me I see all healing as the same. Healing is healing. I am simply changing frequencies at a level of light and information. In each case I am just a vessel for the energy or light. I am "the Facilitator". This for me is no more serious than a headache. It's no less serious than a life threatening road traffic accident. I treat everything the same, with zero judgement.

Sometimes I may facilitate a few healing sessions close together if a patient is riddled with tumours, if necessary, depending on the reaction from the client, but I treat every dis-ease with the same authority. And that is none. It's simply stuck energy in the body, or stuck energy in another space or parallel dimension, one linked to the human being in question, that needs to be moved or shifted.

The emotional cause of Mark's stuff was not taking care of himself. He was putting everyone else before himself and not loving and nurturing his body the way it should have been. Something else I did with Mark was to change his nutrition. I always take a full holistic approach and recommend exercise and nutritional changes when necessary. It's surprising how many people think they know what healthy is, but they are eating far from healthy. Remember, your body is a natural organism and it requires nature to thrive.

Putting man-made, so-called food into your belly, is not going to aid you on your journey, to unlock your greatness and release your full human potential, out into the YOU-Niverse. We will discuss nutrition later on.

I have come to realize that we humans are very much like plants, trees and flowers. We need water, sunlight and oxygen to thrive. Over recent years my entire nutritional way has changed. I am no longer following the programme that was installed into me as a youngster, which consisted of three square meals. I eat, as and when, I want to. The majority of my nutrition comes from light. I will spend time each day sun-gazing and performing some other techniques/ways, which enable your body to metabolize light as nutrition.

It is possible to bring in fifth-dimensional light rays from other worlds or spaces, and your body can metabolize this light as energy. After all we are light. Our human body is an illusion. I eat less food now and feed off of more light. If you ask anyone who has been to one of my workshops, they will tell you that their nutrition completely changes afterwards. This is because I take them so deep in the deep-frequency encoded meditations, and bring so much light through their bodily hologram, that it activates something within them. It activates dormant genetic encodements within their human DNA.

As the observer of Mark's situation I simply created a different reality. He was told there were cysts, growths, blood tests with E-coli and Peritonitis and I simply chose to see it differently – a body containing none of this. I chose to see a perfectly healthy body. Science has proven that the observer affects the observed. It offers us the power of alchemy.

8

In the Eye of the Observer

Star Magic is imaginative and the infinite possibilities that lie within your imagination are, as I just suggested, infinite. Mainstream medicine has its place and there are some wonderful practitioners out there. The medical industry itself, however, has created a reality model that constricts, pigeon-holes and keeps most people suffering, due to the medical grid structure that has been created across this planet.

When a patient goes to see his or her doctor they are asked what the problem is. Once the problem has been highlighted the doctor will re-inforce the issue by prescribing tablets for it, or maybe a set of treatments or even surgery. The doctor is working inside of a system. This system has problems and solutions. The solution is always prescribed, off of the back of the problem. This is dysfunctional as what is being created is more of the problem. Each time a solution is given the problem grows in strength and re-enforces the medical grid system, contained within the Universal Database.

Reality itself is held in the eye of the observer and he or she who is observing a particular situation, interprets it in their own special and unique way. Two people viewing the same situation can both be right in their own minds. Are they both right? Yes, their version of reality is what they perceive.

When it comes to consciousness, everything that is ever thought or felt, is infused into the ether – into the field, the Universal Database. Each time a doctor asks a series of questions to a patient they narrow down the possible causes until it fits into the rule book they were taught at medical school. OK, well you have this and that and you're not sleeping at night so you must have this problem. The patient then believes they have it. If that patient doesn't get better they may go and seek the help of another doctor or human being in the field of alternative medicine.

They may end up seeing several different people, all with a different perspective. Each of these different perspectives is having a major effect on the human being in question. Because the observer affects the observed, creating new realities, the observed becomes completely confused in the realm of possibilities. Why? Because the different diagnoses, from the different doctors, have created different subsets of realities, all within the energy field of the human being in question.

Everyone is thinking logically, inside the parameters of what has been taught. This does not engage your imagination. Your imagination is relegated to the depths of despair, forgotten, because imagination is not in the medical rule book. When you treat symptoms and conditions you never eliminate the cause. Star Magic eliminates the cause, not by eliminating it, but by changing the reality of the observed, through the eye of the observer. In this case me, or you, or whoever is facilitating the Star Magic healing session. Working with Star Magic enables you to create with the very same Star Dust you were originated from. Star Light and Star Dust are the keys.

The reason Star Magic is so powerful is because it steps outside of the confinements of a system. If Star Magic was a system you would be limited by it. Fortunately, it's not. It's an expansive, growing, developing technology that has zero limits. The limits are held within the eye of the observer. What do you think Doctor Jones would say if I told him I could make his patient's tumour disappear with the help of my Unicorn? Well, I did do that at a spiritual fayre. I was engaged in a deep conversation with a lady, whom I didn't know was a doctor. She told me she was, as she slammed my advertising material back down on the table and looked at me like I was completely bonkers.

On the other hand I have had many a client who has shared their experiences with me, with their own doctor. The doctor has embraced the work and told them to carry on as it's clearly working. I have asked many doctors to join me in an interview to talk about energy and Star Magic healing and most have said if they were seen to support it they would lose their job and more importantly their reputation. Why are we not working together? Everything has its place.

When I have a client with some so-called medical condition I never go to work to combat that condition. If I were to do that I would give it power. Instead, using my observation I change the reality surrounding the situation. When I look at a human being in terms of energy, I see wave patterns and particles. When the waves are not flowing correctly I change them. This then manifests in the physical body. You don't need to know what the problem is to take it away.

Observe the energy and the solution will appear.

9

Light Is Fuel –
Activate the Bio-Transducer

Current human genetic science calls 99% of the DNA "junk", because, "we don't know what it all means". In fact, human DNA holds bits of genetic material from every other species on Earth, plus genetic material holographically encoded with the collective experience of all of humanity. And... the experiences of your holographic grid of incarnations, as well as bits of genetic encoding from the sentient species of hundreds, maybe thousands (yes, we are not alone) of ascending planets across multiple local Universes!

Your DNA also holds latent encodements for mutating your physical body into a light dody. A body that metabolizes light as nutrition.

As Star Magic is used to bring in light from other worlds, intelligent light of an extremely high frequency, these Extra-Terrestrial Space Codes, activate a series of these latent encodements by infusing a tone/colour sequence. These newly activated encodements signal your body to begin a mutational change in the DNA, and a profound alteration in the way your cells metabolize energy. This is the beginning of a powerful stream of never ending healing and infinite growth.

We measure light body levels by the ability of your cells to metabolize light. The market for this new cellular activity is the amount of adenosine triphosphate (ATP) in the cells. Before light body activation, the energy for cellular functioning came from an energy production and storage system, which shuttles energy back and forth between adenosine diphosphate (ADP) and adenosine triphosphate (ATP).

ATP is an energy storage compound found in the cells. Within the mitochondria, food is converted into energy for the cells, which is then bound up in the ATP. ATP has a chain of three phosphate groups, which projects out from the molecule. When an ATP molecule loses its outermost phosphate group, it becomes an ADP molecule. The breaking of the chemical bond releases energy for the cell to carry out its functions, such as creating proteins.

ADP can again become ATP by picking up some energy and a phosphate group. ATP and ADP lose and gain phosphate groups to release any stored energy for cellular functioning. This is a closed system of biological energy, ensuring aging and death. No new energy is gained.

When the light body mutation is activated through Star Magic, a series of latent DNA encodements light up and begin to give new directives to cells. One of the first instructions is to tell the cells to recognize light as a new source of energy. Remember we are Star Dust through and through. We are returning to our original natural state.

At first, the cellular consciousness doesn't know what to do with this information. As the cells are bathed in light, the mitochondria (which are very light sensitive) begin to fully absorb this new colour/tonal activation and produce lots of ATP, in bursts. The cells at this stage cannot yet absorb enough light to stabilize the phosphate bond, so the ATP breaks down very rapidly into ADP, and cellular metabolism is dramatically speeded up. Accumulated toxins, old traumas, and stored thoughts and emotions begin to flush from the physical body, and create cold or flu-like symptoms.

The physical form in its old manner has separated brain functioning into right and left hemisphere functions. Also, the pineal gland and pituitary glands are atrophied – about the size of a pea rather than a walnut. On activation, brain chemistry begins to change and to produce new synapses.

Everything that happens at this stage is very centred in the physical body. It's beginning to open up into what I call a "bio-transducer system". Your body was designed to decode and work with higher light energies/frequencies as well as transmit these energies/frequencies to the planet. As part of the game of separation, these functions atrophied. The magnification of the physical senses is the first sign of the awakening of your body as a bio-transducer.

Each cell of your body, once you start to utilize the light absorption technique I will share with you, has light focused directly into them, through the channelled network of light (CNL). The channelled network of light is a grid system that surrounds your body and connects you to everything in this Universe. There are streams of light coming out from your body in all directions. Once you start to use Star Magic you will see this grid. It is phenomenal. This grid gives you access to so much knowledge.

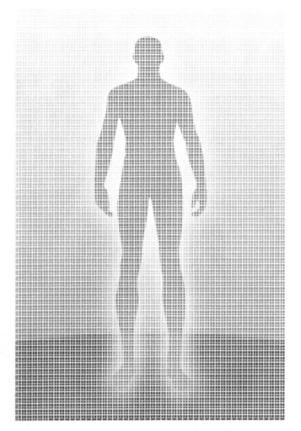

1. The grid of light beams coming in from all directions

The picture is not entirely accurate. If all the streams of light that enter the human body were drawn you wouldn't actually see the body. There really is that much light. You really are a pattern of light with no physical form. There are also other patterns of light surrounding the human body that look like shapes and geometric patterns. Your human field of light is breathtaking. We will discuss parts of the light body structure later on.

The mitochondria usually recognize this light as food, and produce more ATP. Because the cell is receiving light as usable energy, less of the ATP turns into ADP. As light is fed from source, from the stars, through the CNL, into the cellular spin points within your body and around your body, the spin points produce sound and light frequencies which change the atomic spin of the cell's molecules, especially in the hydrogen atoms.

As the atomic spin in the ATP molecule increases, a new functioning emerges. The three phosphate groups forming the stalk of the ATP molecule begin to act like an antenna for undifferentiated light, and the symmetrical head of the molecule acts like a prism, breaking down the light into subtle colour spectrums, usable by the dormant DNA encodements.

Before your light body is activated, the ribonucleic acid (RNA) in the cells acted as a one-way messenger. It carried directives from the active 7% of the DNA (the encodements waiting for instruction) to other parts of the cell for execution – such as what proteins to synthesize. The RNA becomes a two-way messenger! Now it takes light, broken down into usable colour frequencies by the ATP antenna/prism, back into the DNA strands. The dormant genetic encodements gradually awaken as you begin to bring in more light and give their information to the RNA, which transmits it to the rest of the cell.

It is much like CD laser technologies on Earth. An enormous amount of information can be stored on one disk. Imagine that a vast amount can be stored in a colour range of red and vast amounts of data can be stored in the green spectrum. A red laser beam is run across the disk and all the red information is now available to be read, but you still know nothing about what is stored in the green spectrum. You then run a green laser beam over the disk and then all of the information is made available. There are not just two colour spectrums, there are many.

The light colour frequencies "read" the DNA in much the same way. Until the colour spectrum is transmitted, you have no idea what's in there. Each light body level has its own colour/tonal signature. In this way, Spirit achieves the gradual mutation of the physical body. There are a number of levels you go through. The more you utilize Star Magic, the more you will remember, and the more powerful you will become.

The one-way DNA to RNA information transfer and the ATP to ADP energy cycle were closed systems, ensuring entropy. Nothing could change, except to decay. With light body activation, new, fully open systems can develop, making infinite energy and infinite information available to the body. A dialogue between your physical body and Spirit opens up a brand new and exciting world for you. It's not easy. It requires effort. Are you prepared to do what is necessary to light up your world?

Basic Light Absorption Way

To kick-start you on the way to nourishing your own body with light I want to share this easy to use and very powerful light absorption way with you:

Stand outside and look up towards the sky. Place your thumbs together and your forefingers together and create a triangular prism. Hold that over your heart, close your eyes and see in your mind's eye the Great Central Sun. This is a sun behind the sun, the centre of our Universe. Imagine it as a bright white light with an electric blue, almost transparent coat. The Central Sun is a level of consciousness that exists as a white and blue ball of light. It carries light from the fifth world. Focus and see this sun shining brightly out in space. You don't need to know exactly where it is. Know that it is everywhere.

The Great Central Sun is the point of integration of the Spirit/Matter Cosmos, and the Origin of all physical-spiritual creation. The sun behind the sun is the Spiritual cause behind the physical effect we see as our own physical sun and all other stars and star systems, seen or unseen, including the Great Central Sun.

With your intention you will summon this light as everything is in the same place or space always. See a stream of brilliant pure white crystalline energy, flowing from this sun, in through your triangular prism, and into your body.

Still your mind and do this exercise from anywhere between ten and twenty minutes. You will feel it. You will feel full. Your stomach will feel full and your body will feel nourished. If it's cloudy it doesn't matter. We are talking on a level of super-consciousness. Consciousness can effortlessly travel through every hard man-made material (as everything is conscious-ness), so to travel through a few clouds is also effortless. You could even do this from within your home. I just prefer to go outside. I recommend doing this, every day. You may notice instant results, as I did, or it may take a little longer. Be patient and keep doing it.

To be a Star Magic Facilitator and learn the way of the force, you must learn or remember to be like a plant, a flower or a tree. A tree needs water, light and oxygen. You and I are no different. The more you work with Star Magic the less you will eat, and that which you do eat will be pure.

10

The Facilitator

Let me make something very clear. I am no different from you. We are all human beings cut from the same cloth, created by the very same energy. We are all divine beings, manifested into human form, and each one of us carries the potential to be a Star Magic Facilitator. You can do everything that I can do. As you know, there was a time when I hadn't remembered anything, which I am sharing in this book, and yet, I remembered all that I am sharing and much more.

I will continue to remember more and enhance Soul Technology, creating more advanced versions of human potential. The deeper you journey, the more there is to unlock, and re-discover. It's extremely exciting to think where Star Magic will take us in the near now. It will re-shape and re-mould the medical industry, the travel industry (local and YOU-Niversal), communication, the food industry and will totally transform the vibration on this planet.

My mission is to heal one billion people. It starts with you. You are powerful and you must know this. I am not sharing this information so you can read and think well, "Jerry may be able to do it but it doesn't mean I can." No! You are no different from me, and my plan is to inspire you to journey, and empower you to heal yourself and then use these ways to heal others.

If you work with energy already, you can use Star Magic to elevate your skills. Reiki practitioners often come to me for healing, as my reputation for helping existing practitioners become more powerful energy healers, has grown rapidly. People tell me how their clients feel the frequencies pouring from their bodies. Practitioners seem to be more aware and function at a higher capacity after utilizing Star Magic.

Star Magic works on such a deep level, that it unblocks and releases anything that is holding a human being back, and when those blocks are released the light and energy flows freely. But it doesn't just flow freely. It ignites the light of your Star Seed nature and crystallizes the abilities that have been hidden beneath your human appearance for a long, long time.

People often say to me that they are a Reiki Master and have been doing Reiki for twenty-five years, but they have never experienced anything like Star

Magic. It really is a different level. Other Healing modalities have taken us so far in this world, which is incredible. They paved the way and started the healing ball rolling. Now it's time to raise the bar.

I never in my wildest dreams expected Star Magic to have the kind of effect on people that it has. I am just so grateful that I can pass this information on, and have such a positive effect on the human race. We all have certain limiting beliefs that stop us from achieving our highest potential. Star Magic will clear these. Once you open your mind, fully, there are no limitations, just infinite possibilities.

After Star Magic has worked its way into your cells, and removed any deep-rooted pain, your energy and light frequencies will flow in ways I cannot describe with words. It's experiential. You have the power to be a Star Magic Facilitator. I can offer you suggestions but you must walk the path. No one can do it for you. Dedication and commitment to unravel your personal mystery is required.

You have the power of alchemy. You can turn water into wine or copper into gold. All is possible because all is energy. Change your perception and you will change your world. As you read through the healing techniques, which I prefer to call "ways" don't try and be like me. Don't copy me. I am merely offering suggestions on how to facilitate healing. Use your imagination and interpret reality in your own special and unique way.

Remember Star Magic is not a system. It's not a formula or a programme. It's a non-systematical way of knowing. Playfulness, fun, exploration within the use of your imagination, are mission-critical. Be rigid and you are limited. Try and be like me and you are limiting your own power. You may be able to use Star Magic in a much better way than me. Open yourself fully to all that is and all that it is not.

When I drop into my heart to heal, something we will discuss later, I connect with the Universal Database and the Quantum World opens up to me. Nothing about it is logical and trust is the key. Trust that what you see is there to serve you in healing the human being in question.

I had a lady with Irritable Bowel Syndrome and was a few minutes into the healing. I saw in my vision – which is like a computer game when I drop into my healing zone – an old truck engine with a red misty light or energy within it. I instantly knew that the engine, with all its pipes, tubes and components were the ladies bowels. The red energy was what was causing the issue. I visualized white light coming into the engine and rinsing and cleaning it out. I did this until there was no more red misty light left.

The lady's Irritable Bowel Syndrome cleared immediately. I didn't plan on making this happen. I simply dropped into the healing zone. Here I let the journey begin. When you set out on a journey you haven't travelled before you don't imagine the roads will be a certain way. Instead, you simply travel them. They unfold as you move. On a dark night you can only ever see just in front of your headlights. Do you worry that the road beyond this won't open up? No! You simply keep travelling and know that it will.

When it comes to healing, drop into the zone and be ready for an adventure.

11

Slow Motion

I have been in several car accidents in my life. I will share another one with you now. It was early evening on Boxing Day - Boxing Day always seems to be eventful for me. I was driving home thinking to myself, "I can't wait to see Laura and the kids", then crunch… a taxi driver who was speeding came straight across the cross-roads without stopping and hit my passenger side door. I only know the full story of what happened next because the driver behind told me afterwards.

Once the taxi hit my car, its power combined with my forward momentum took me straight into a lamp post, my head went through the windscreen, my car rebounded off the lamp post and span about thirty metres up the road. During the spin I actually came to. I must have been knocked out for a split second and then regained consciousness. I saw a wall coming towards me and I thought to myself, "My passenger door is crumpled, the front end of the car is crushed and if I hit the wall and the engine blows up I will be trapped."

The time it took from waking up to getting to the wall must have been a second, maybe two. Everything slowed down for me though. I entered a completely different reality. I had the thoughts about the wall, the passenger door and the front of the car and being trapped and then jumping from the car. It happened so slowly though. It felt like I had enough time to boil the kettle, drink a cup of tea and leisurely get out from the car, which I did. Not the cup of tea part but the leisurely part yes.

I climbed up out of the car, got out of the way and then the car smashed into the wall. The neighbours that came outside said it sounded like a bomb went off. This reality that I went into during this accident is a reality that we can step between whenever we like. I enter this version of reality every time I facilitate a healing. Explaining it using the accident, is the best way I can describe it. Maybe that is why I had it?

I will share with you another story surrounding this accident (incident is a better way to describe it as I don't feel there are any accidents), which is important. The next day my right eye was filling up with blood and it felt as though someone was stepping on my eyeball and it was about to be squashed like a grape.

I decided to see a local doctor – purely because of this accident – as I never go. This is what she said: *"I think you need to toughen up Mr Sargeant."* I walked out of there laughing. A little annoyed but I found it funny that this is what I was hearing.

I went to Accident and Emergency (A&E) and had a scan. They said there was a crack in my eye socket and my nerves were being pinched in between the crack. This is what was causing the pain. They said they would need to observe me. I realized that coming to the hospital and the doctor was a waste of time, in this scenario. So I decided to see what I could do myself. I probably should have just sorted it myself but everyone was saying: *"Jerry, this is your brain; you should really go and get it checked out."* So I did.

Anyway, that evening I sat down, dropped into my heart, my healing zone and took an imaginary tube. Well, in the reality that I created it wasn't imaginary. I stuck this tube into the side of my head. I went through my right temple and I pushed it in until the other end of the tube was just behind my right eyeball. I then sucked on the tube to siphon out the blood. I left it to run into my imaginary, but very real bucket, in the fourth dimension.

As the blood was running out I used my hands to re-correct the eye socket and release the nerve. I then meditated and went to bed. When I woke up in the morning there was no blood in my eye. It was completely clear, the pain had gone and I felt brand new. This just goes to show the power of imagination with focused intent. And, a little sprinkle of love, knowing and of course light.

All I did was create a new reality and merge/quantum entangle the two together.

12

Intrinsic Value

When you start to work with Star Magic, it is fair to say, that you may still and probably will, believe. You will believe, possibly, in religion, other people, ideas, ways of handling certain situations, maybe a political party and you may or may not believe in yourself.

I actually encourage you to not believe in yourself. I encourage you to not believe in anything. Stop believing in a religion, faith, a family member, friend or community. Don't believe in any ideas. Don't believe in anything anyone ever tells you and certainly don't believe in me, or the information in this book. Don't believe the thoughts that are inside of your own head. Make a pact from here on in that you will not believe in anything. If you can't do that just yet, then that is OK. Keep reading.

Belief systems are based on your thoughts. You cannot think Star Magic. You have to transcend thinking, move from your left to right brain and work intuitively. You have to know Star Magic. When you know something you know it. Nothing can supercede what you know. A belief is different. Knowing trumps believing, every single time. When you know you know. It's a given.

We may encourage our children to believe in themselves. *"Come on son, you can do it."* Why do they believe they can do it? Whatever that "it" may be. They use their thoughts to convince themselves that they can do it. And yes, it often works. Maybe they convince themselves that they can do it, maybe, because out of the fear of not being able to do it. Is that productive? Well, it can be a step in the right direction. Believing can be a stepping stone towards knowing. It's like an athlete that runs a race. They build up to a certain time. After a while they know that they can achieve this time as they have achieved it so often. They don't second-guess. They know their own ability.

So, when it comes to knowing oneself, believing can be a stepping stone. Believing in your religion, your community or family is a different matter though. When we believe in a religion or a community we hand our power over to whatever it is that we believe in. Why would we do that? Why would we do that when we are the technology? We are the power! We are Star Dust! We are Star Magic!

When we are a part of a community or a group, we feel powerful. What happens when we leave that group? Most people will not leave a group or a community, once they are in it, because of the fear of being alone, being ostracized, being fearful of losing their power.

It's OK to be a part of a community but you must not hand your power over in the process. You must know that if you leave that community, your power will not change. *You carry an intrinsic value. That value is you.* Not you and your business partner…. You and your husband or wife…. You and your church…. **You** are the power. (It's like money. If you burn a twenty pound note it's then worth nothing. If you take a gold coin, melt it down and split it into five pieces, the total value of those five pieces will be the same as when the coin was whole. Gold carries an intrinsic value.)

You must *know* this. I cannot give you this. No one can. It must come from a self-realization that you control how you think, your emotional responses to life situations, your ability to handle and overcome every challenge, and in doing so, you use a basic form of alchemy. The power of perception. What do I mean? Turning obstacles into opportunities by seeing things in a certain way.

Was Jesus any different from you? No, he simply knew the truth. Nothing more. Nothing less. Jesus understood Star Magic – like many before and many after, he knew himself. He knew he was a Star Seed created from Star Dust and in knowing so he knew his own intrinsic value.

Feel life. Don't think your way through it. Get in touch with your feminine side. Yes, men, that includes you too. I am not saying never to think, don't get me wrong. In this human world it can be useful, especially if you want to meet someone at 3pm. When Star Magic is concerned it has to be felt. You must know it. You have to know it to unlock its full potential. As long as you believe in it you will be limited. You may still get some results but the full force, the full power of Star Magic, will not flow freely through your veins.

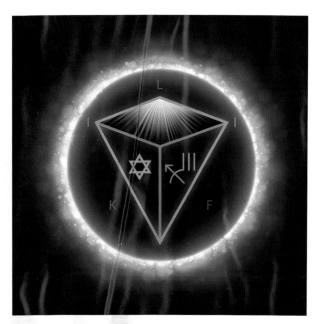

Healing Magic symbol (p. 24)

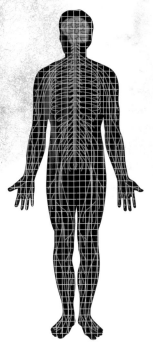

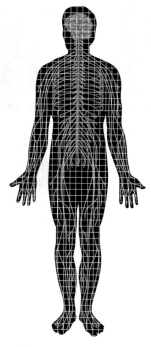

10. Hologram with nervous system
before the healing – red (p.82)

11. Hologram with nervous system
after the healing – green (p.82)

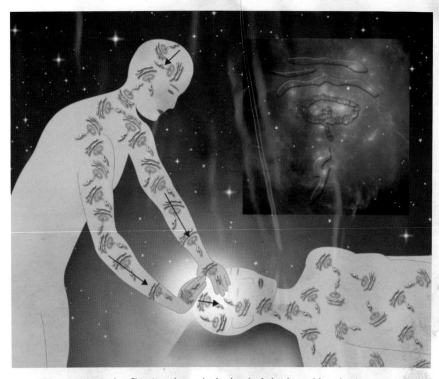

22. Codes flowing through the healer's body and hands via
the crown chakra into the client's body (p.102)

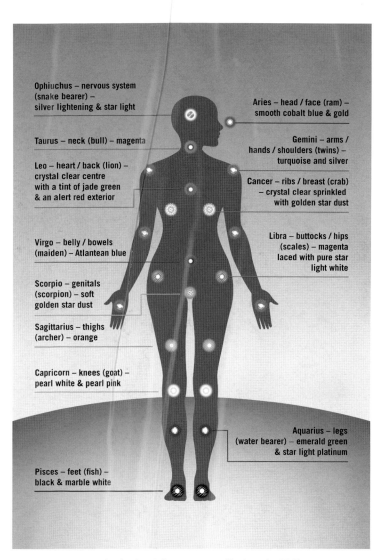

Ophiuchus – nervous system
(snake bearer) –
silver lightening & star light

Aries – head / face (ram) –
smooth cobalt blue & gold

Taurus – neck (bull) – magenta

Gemini – arms /
hands / shoulders (twins) –
turquoise and silver

Leo – heart / back (lion) –
crystal clear centre
with a tint of jade green
& an alert red exterior

Cancer – ribs / breast (crab)
– crystal clear sprinkled
with golden star dust

Virgo – belly / bowels
(maiden) – Atlantean blue

Libra – buttocks / hips
(scales) – magenta
laced with pure star
light white

Scorpio – genitals
(scorpion) – soft
golden star dust

Sagittarius – thighs
(archer) – orange

Capricorn – knees (goat) –
pearl white & pearl pink

Aquarius – legs
(water bearer) – emerald green
& star light platinum

Pisces – feet (fish) –
black & marble white

57. The body with star constellations (p. 215)

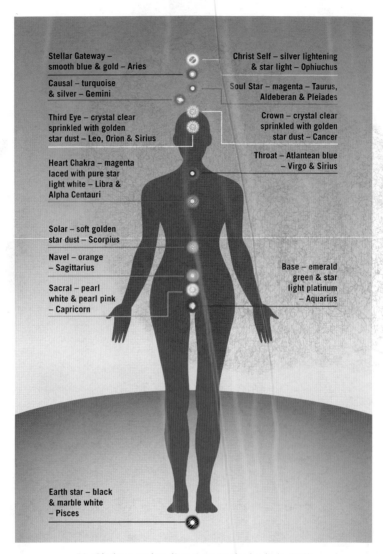

Stellar Gateway –
smooth blue & gold – Aries

Causal – turquoise
& silver – Gemini

Third Eye – crystal clear
sprinkled with golden
star dust – Leo, Orion & Sirius

Heart Chakra – magenta
laced with pure star
light white – Libra &
Alpha Centauri

Solar – soft golden
star dust – Scorpius

Navel – orange
– Sagittarius

Sacral – pearl
white & pearl pink
– Capricorn

Christ Self – silver lightening
& star light – Ophiuchus

Soul Star – magenta – Taurus,
Aldeberan & Pleiades

Crown – crystal clear
sprinkled with golden
star dust – Cancer

Throat – Atlantean blue
– Virgo & Sirius

Base – emerald
green & star
light platinum
– Aquarius

Earth star – black
& marble white
– Pisces

58. Chakras and zodiac signs in the body (p. 217)

PART 3

13

Temperature Control & the
Nerve Fibre Building Process

Later on in this book I will discuss sound and how it can be useful for activating the Third Eye. When it comes to building your life force, chi, prana, your energy or light flow, however, it's not effective, even though some healing modalities teach this. There are techniques that teach people to bring energy into certain parts of the body in particular, and also to use heat. Firstly, remember we are working with light, with information. Secondly know that we are not running energy. We are changing patterns of light or patterns of information.

When it comes to Star Magic, no part of my body is hot. I have trained it to be this way. Occasionally my hands will emit a little warmth but at the same time if you were to touch my hands they would be ice-cold. My hands also vibrate when I am scanning the holographic blueprint of a human being. They vibrate at a place I need to bring my awareness into.

Regardless of what anyone tells you or what you have read, the only way to truly know is to experience. I want you to experience temperature control within your own body.

Healing is more effective when the body is cool. The light and energy can flow more freely and there are no side effects, for the human being facilitating the healing process. When your body is warm, it's out of balance. When you focus on bringing energy/light into certain parts of your body and neglecting others, you are out of balance.

Being out of balance can result in different side effects. They are unhealthy. You can experience vertigo, organ pains, muscle pain, headaches, pins and needles and sickness. It's not pleasant. It's ineffective to facilitate a healing and get ill yourself in the process.

If you are a healer and have been taught that heat is good, and you are getting some results, which you still can do, then try for a change bringing your own body temperature down and see what results you get then. You will be amazed.

When you are facilitating the healing of someone, they may feel heat, or cold, and both are OK. It means healing is taking place. It's different for the person being healed than for the healer. The healer wants to maintain a nice cool temperature flow for two reasons – safety and effectiveness. It's also mission-critical to treat your entire body as a healing vessel, not just certain parts of it. We are not mechanical, we are natural.

Within your body you have approximately forty-five miles of electrical wiring or nerve fibres. They spread throughout your entire body. The secret to powerful energy/light is to build up the entire nervous system. You have to build it up throughout the entire body. If you try to pocket light and energy in certain areas, like your hands, you are limiting yourself.

To fully experience the power of Star Magic, you must build up your entire nervous system, and once you do, learn to regulate the temperature of the energy flow throughout your body. Once you do this you fully activate the CNL or light grid system throughout and extending beyond your entire body, enabling you to work on a level of light and information much more easily.

To build up the nervous system you need to use light. You use your awareness to tune into the nervous system and feel the light energy flow. Then, by bringing in more light, you can increase the flow, strengthen the system and increase the bandwidth, which in turn, will enable more light to flow throughout the entire nervous system, in turn allowing more information to flow through it. Remember light is information.

As the bandwidth of the nervous system grows and strengthens, so does the amount of light/energy you can use, and the volume of information contained within the light can be increased. You can also add, through your intention, more information to this light. You will understand this when we discuss Star Magic Codes of Consciousness later on.

There is said to be four thousand nerve fibres in your hands and around four hundred in your feet. Wouldn't it be great to have four thousand in your feet too? Imagine if you had a high volume of nerve fibres running throughout your entire system, and you could control and direct the flow of light through them all. Well, soon you will. And you are going to be able to control the temperature at the same time. Your body will have its own built-in air conditioning unit.

Nerve Fibre Building Process

Remember you cannot push light or energy around your body. Energy has to flow and light is everywhere. You can control this flow but never by force. By forcing light or running energy you will experience the same symptoms as using too much heat. When you overload your system in one area, it's too much electricity in that area, so the nerve fibre building process must be executed throughout the entire body. It's easy to feel energy in your hands so most people work with their hands.

When your entire system is built effectively, light pours from all parts of your body evenly, through the ether, carrying information necessary for healing, and into the energy field or body, of the human being you are facilitating the healing of.

Bio-photons, which are units of light, collect between the nerve fibres.

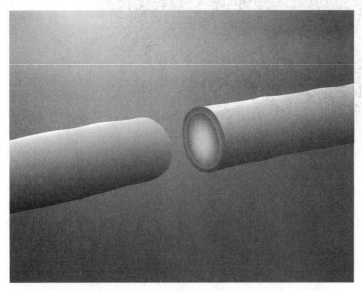

2. Nerve fibres without the biophotons

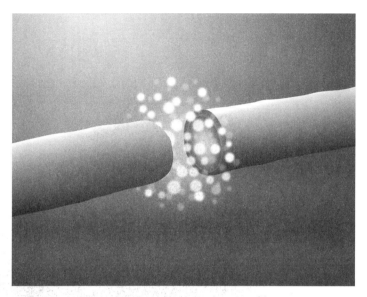

3. Biophotons in between the nerve fibres

To build your nervous system into one complete and powerful unit, you will need to use your imagination, your intention and your awareness. Once your Third Eye is activated properly (which we will discuss later on), you will be able to see what is happening, but until then these three ingredients are crucial. You will also need to trust and know. Before you start this process, it's good to have an idea of what the nervous system looks like.

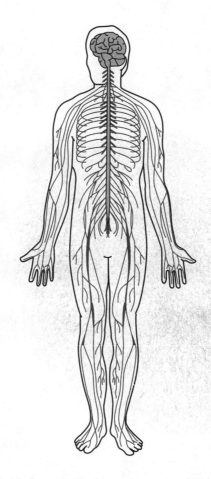

4. A hologram with the nervous system inside

You can start by bringing in light through the top of your head and see it flow throughout your nerve fibres. Just have your awareness over the nerve fibres inside your face and head. Use your imagination and see the light flow around with your intention. Tell it where to flow. Command/intend it but don't force it. *Remember your body responds to your intention.* Once you feel/ see or know the light has spread throughout each nerve fibre, you can stop.

You can then repeat the process with your neck. Then, with your shoulders and chest. Next, your back and arms. Then, your stomach area. Then, your hips and buttocks. Now your legs, and finally your feet. Once the light is flowing through the entire system you can stop. Once you see this light flowing through your entire nervous system, you are ready to start building it – slowly!

23-Day Programme

Below I give you a phased 23-day way for you to build up and strengthen your nervous system. Do this and you will enhance your ability to heal as well as feel happier, stronger and lighter in your vibration.

DAYS 1-5 Spend 15 minutes repeating the above process. By the end of the five days you should be able to activate your entire nervous system, with light, at once. See this light as a white colour. If it takes you longer than five days, that is perfectly OK.

DAY 6 Repeat as above. Then with your imagination and intention see the nerve fibres start to expand and grow thicker, just inside your head. The entire process should take no longer than fifteen minutes. Every day; no longer than fifteen minutes.

DAY 7 Repeat as above adding the next body part, your neck.

DAY 8 Repeat as above adding the next body parts, your shoulders and chest.

DAY 9 Repeat as above adding the next body part, your back and arms.

DAY 10 Repeat as above adding the next body part, your stomach area.

DAY 11 Repeat as above adding the next body part, your hips and buttocks.

DAY 12 Repeat as above adding the next body part, your legs.

DAY 13 Repeat as above adding the next body part, your feet.

DAY 14-21 Repeat the expansion process including every body part at once. Don't force anything. You will see the nervous system gradually expand and more energy will flow through it. Keep bringing the light in, and it will naturally happen, through using your intention and imagination. Feel the process with your awareness. When you come back to this, after your Third Eye is open and functioning, you will see it clearly.

DAY 22 Bring the light into your body and throughout your entire nervous system. See or feel (both maybe) the light flowing through. Now, start to project your energy evenly from your nervous system outwards. See or feel (maybe both) it expand, evenly in all directions. The aim of this exercise is to see light projecting from your entire body, outwards. As you get used to doing this, your body's light will naturally start doing this during the healing process, when you are facilitating the healings of others. Your body has this entire electrical system, you have to hone it. Do this until it feels like you should stop!

DAY 23 Expand it further. Do this every day until you can fill a room with your light in a heartbeat.

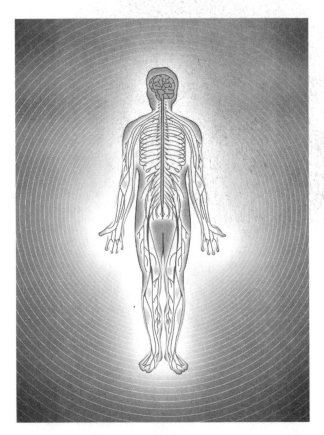

5. Energy from nervous system projecting
throughout the entire room

At my Star Magic Training Experiences, where I facilitate the remembering of Star Magic with people, and share everything I know I get people to do this exercise. When everyone does this at once it feels like I am out at sea and the water is rough. The expansion of light and energy takes me off of my feet.

From here on in, spend fifteen minutes every day bringing light through your nervous system. See it flow and feel it flow. Start to understand how it flows. See and feel the patterns, the geometry. Watch it expand and ensure it expands evenly and that you can project this energy at will, evenly, through all areas of your body. If one area seems to be weaker than others, put your intention forward to strengthen it. But never force it. Increase the size of the individual nerve fibres.

Remember, throughout this entire process, drop down into your heart space. Bring your awareness there. Your awareness can be in as many places at once as you wish.

Regulating the Temperature

You want your body to remain cool. Think cool and you will be cool. It really is that easy. You will need to have your awareness scanning or feeling your entire body, as you are facilitating the healing. If it feels as though it's getting hot just think ice, think cool. Imagine a cool breeze flowing through your body. You don't want it to be as cold as ice, because it may take your intention away from the healing, as you will be too cold, but thinking ice, can quickly cool you down.

Once you have started to see and feel your body becoming cooler, set your intention to maintain the temperature that feels cool for you. You will get to know your body through your awareness, and you will soon realize if it's too hot, as you may experience some of the side effects such as headaches, vertigo, pins and needles, aching organs etc.

You can see the flow of energy throughout your own body as a cool blue colour. This will help in keeping it cool. See the energy as red on the other hand, which is often associated with fire and heat, and you will get hot.

Once your nervous system is fully activated and you can regulate the light energy flow at a cool temperature, you will be able to project your energy effortlessly and powerfully, manipulating realities with your own energy field, light field or CNL.

That means with no effort at all. *That is the key to Star Magic.* You create an environment where it all happens for you. You really do become a pure vessel. You truly facilitate without action. As you progress through the basic, intermediate and onto the advanced healing ways, all of this will become clear to you.

14

Preparing for Facilitation

Preparation for the facilitation of a healing session is more important than the healing session itself. If you don't prepare properly, it's less effective. It's the same with everything in life, preparation is mission-critical. The more you work with Star Magic, the more you will understand why.

So how do I prepare for a healing session? Whether it's at distance or when I am in the same room, working privately, or with a large group, the preparation process is always the same. The healing session itself, once started, changes from human being to human being and we will discuss that separately.

Before a distance healing session, I will ask for a photo of the human being that requires healing. I like to connect through the eyes. It's not a necessity, as I have facilitated healings without a photo, but the connection, for me personally, seems to be better when I have a photo.

The first thing I will do is slow my heart rate down and alter my state; an altered state of consciousness. I will drop into my heart. I will take nice long deep breaths for a minute or so. It used to take several minutes to alter my state of consciousness, through deep breathing, and now it happens much faster. Once my heart rate drops I drop into a state, somewhere between being asleep, and being awake. When people are in deep meditation they are said to be in the Theta State. It's where most people are when they are drifting off to sleep. It's a great state for harnessing your creativity. It's why so many incredible ideas come in meditation.

The Delta State is the next level. Your brain waves are even slower. This is the state where you can bring your light from your body and travel. However, we are only going to dabble in that in this book. In the Delta State you enter the realms of deep unconscious and intuitive insight. It's very easy to drift off to sleep once you get to this stage, and so the trick is to enter these realms somewhere between Theta and Delta and at the same time remain alert and functional. This takes practise.

A great way to do this is to fill a glass right to the top (maybe use plastic to start) with water and sit in a chair. Hold the glass of water in your hands, and start to breathe deeply. You can have your eyes open or closed. Breathe deeply, and slow your heart rate down, and you will feel your state change as you drop down though the levels and come into your centre, your heart space. The aim is to be able to stay in this altered state of consciousness, where intuitive insight comes to you, without spilling the water. You will get wet a few times and that's OK. Practise makes perfect.

As I am breathing and slowing my heart rate down, I will be calling on support from my personal team of spirit guides, and also what I refer to as the Star Team. I will introduce you to the Star Team later on, because once you start to use Star Magic, to help others heal, the Star Team will perform certain roles/miracles. You can use the Star Team to facilitate your own healing, but that is more advanced. You must master the basics first. Remember that advanced doesn't mean harder.

Once I have called upon my personal Spirit Guides/Light Beings I will set my intention. My intention would be to facilitate the healing of "Jon Jones". To infuse Jon Jones's being with Star Magic Codes of Consciousness, I would use a certain code or frequencies for that particular healing – if I had a specific focus. I will share some of the Star Magic Codes of Consciousness later and how you can use them to re-write the software, or change the programme, in someone's biological computer: their brain.

By using a Star Magic code or frequency you can still enter the sea of infinite possibilities. Having a specific focus in this way does not limit you. It's different from setting a clear and outright intention. You can use a code or not – either way it's good to ask to be shown what you don't know to facilitate the healing. Using what you do know limits you to what you know. Magic and miracles lie within the unknown.

Once I have called upon a certain code and asked to be shown what I don't know, I will infuse the healing with compassion, purity, divinity, mastery, healing and unconditional love. I will then open my heart chakra fully (with my intention, feeling and or Third Eye sight) as I drop down into my altered state of consciousness. I will then bring myself into the other human being's space, to commence the facilitation.

Sometimes I will do the healing there, in their space, and other times I will bring them back into my space, or take them to another location. I never know until I start. The light/energy dictates how the healing unfolds. Star Magic is flexible and the light/energy always knows what is best, so you must learn to feel and trust the light. Once you enter this state of consciousness it all becomes clear.

Then information starts to appear for me. I either feel it, see it or know it. Once this happens the light begins to flow and move. You can see it. It's beautiful. I then observe, move and manipulate the frequencies. I de-construct and re-construct the human being's energetic blueprint. When using specific Star Magic Codes of Consciousness (which isn't always the case) I will create a Star Magic Symbol, and then write the code into the symbol. This causes the flow of energy, and ensures that this particular energy or light flow contains specific information.

Now when this happens I will let the light containing Star Magic Codes of Consciousness work of its own accord. I know it's taking place. I then bring another element of my awareness back to the open space of conscious play. I then ensure that the healing is not limited to what the Star Magic Code of Consciousness contains. The more you play the easier it happens. It's important that you don't just use a code. The code is powerful but limited inside the symbol. Use the code when necessary but play in the field of possibility and change.

All of the ways I share with you may seem that they are in some kind of order. They are not. As you begin to remember Star Magic, you will realize that nothing has an order. It's flexible. It's non-systematical. Remember these ways, start to use them, and you will see that they take on a life of their own, as they light up your world.

When a client books a healing session with me, they often experience the healing before the actual date and time of the healing. Remember everything is *now* and once someone engages with me and I commit to them, it's all now. The time of our healing is now. It's all now, so the energies, the light, starts working on some level. It's important (if you are a healer) you let your clients know that they may experience some emotions and change prior to the healing.

It happens on my workshops. Once people commit and book their ticket they often go on an emotional roller coaster. Fear comes up, tears flow like rivers and I get phone calls in the office asking: *"Is this normal?"* People say, *"I am not sure if I should come at the weekend."*

Everyone always does come and it's the best move they ever made. You see, what happens is the ego can kick in. It's in fear of these old non-serving patterns being released, which will, in turn, harness the ego's illusory identity. It panics and therefore fear can kick in.

The ego is ever so cunning and it will pull out every trick in the "preserve my identity" book to keep you stagnant, living small and in fear of the future, or held back by the residue of the non-existent past. Always explain to your clients what can happen once they book a healing session or once they book onto a workshop (if you run one).

15

Holographic Blueprints

Everything that you read from here on in is how I interpret reality inside the healing zone. This is a great place for you to start and it will open your mind to what the imagination can achieve or co-create. From there let your own imagination run wild. The wilder the better. The freer it is the more powerful it will become. Remember, don't aim to be like me. Be your own unique version of reality and co-create miracles with your beauty and conscious intelligence.

I want to make something very clear. Star Magic is fun. You can play with it. The minute you are serious with Star Magic, it stops flowing. The moment you lose sight that the energy and light does the work and that you are actually doing something, other than having a fun, playful and imaginative experience, it will cease. You are just a vessel. The more fun you have with this and the more you let your imagination run wild, trusting in all that you see and feel, the stronger this will work.

Most of the time, people tell me that they have this or that ailment, or dis-ease, and so my focus is to hone in on that and take a look, to view the body on an energetic and a physical level. Ninety percent of the time I look at the energy first, and the physical second. If someone doesn't tell me what is wrong, I will usually pick it up in the energy field. I don't always know exactly what the physical issue is, but in terms of energy, or an energetic blockage, it is very clear. I know that if I remove the blockage or create a different reality, I can create an environment whereby someone can heal.

If I am going to facilitate your healing, and your name is Sally Smith, then once I have looked at your photo I will bring up a holographic blueprint of your body. The blueprints that appear for me look very much like the picture of this hologram on the next page.

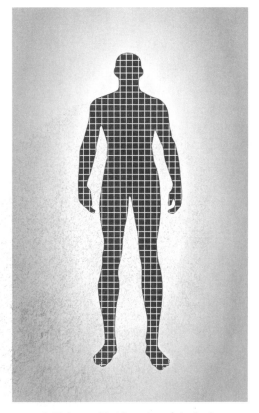

6. Holographic blueprint of the body

Energy Blockages

When I look at this hologram I see it in a variety of different ways. If I am looking for energy blockages, I will see the hologram laid over a blue background. The body will be black with a white energetic grid system throughout, and the energy blockages will show up as white misty particles in areas, and I know I need to clear it. I will clear it by running my hands through it, using my fingers like a comb. The energy will disperse and move back into alignment within the energetic grid system. If it's not geometrical then you know something is amiss.

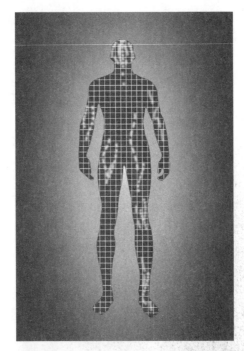

7. How the hologram looks before the healing

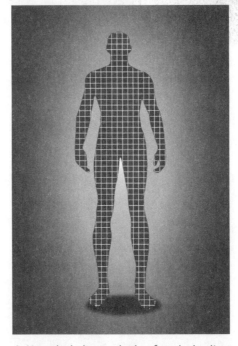

8. How the hologram looks after the healing

The majority of the time, once I have manipulated the energy and moved it back into alignment, the healing will take place. Sometimes however, we need to go deeper.

Organs

When a client tells me they have an issue with a particular organ, whether it's a heart condition, a cyst in the colon or a tumour in the liver, I will see the hologram on a green background, such as in the picture below.

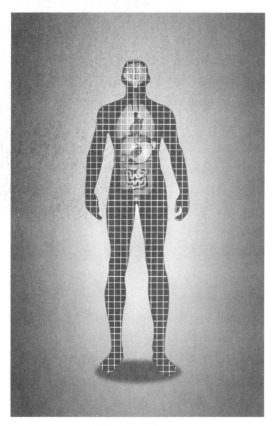

9. Hologram with organs

The organs will look vivid and feel wet, just how they would be inside the body. I will then do what is necessary to facilitate the healing. I will discuss different visualization ways to create healing on another human being in the next chapter and further into the book.

Nervous System

When I am working on the nervous system, I see the holographic blueprint on a white background and the nervous system shows up as red, and then turns to green, once it is healed (see also color insert).

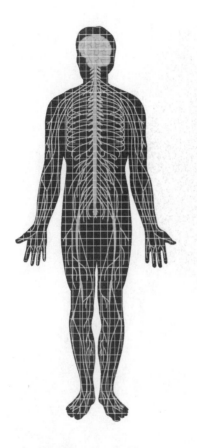 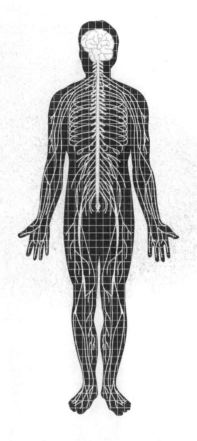

10. Hologram with nervous system before the healing (red)

11. Hologram with nervous system after the healing (green)

Sometimes I may go in to facilitate a healing and the hologram is on a green background because I am working on the organs, and in my mind it will flash to a white background, so I know that the nervous system needs work as well. When you are open and start to work with Star Magic, the energy goes to work for you. It gets easier and easier. It tells you what to do. All you have to do is listen or observe. It's like switching frequencies on a radio station. I go from one channel to the next to listen in. Or in this case see, or feel in.

I will work on the nervous system in neurological cases, when a client has an injury to a limb or joint, is in a coma or has some form of disability. I find that in certain cases of autism, the nervous system plays a vital role. There are cases whereby I work on the nervous system and am not sure exactly why I am doing this. But again, it comes down to trust. This is not a logical experiment. We are working with infinite intelligence and the intelligence knows exactly what has to be done. Remember, I am just the Facilitator. I don't second-guess. I follow my intuition and it's always for the greatest growth of everyone involved.

Skeletal & Aura

When I am working on any part of the skeletal structure I will see the hologram on a black background. The skeletal structure shows up white and the areas that need work either look like cracks, resembling broken bones or fuzzy white energy over the parts that need attention.

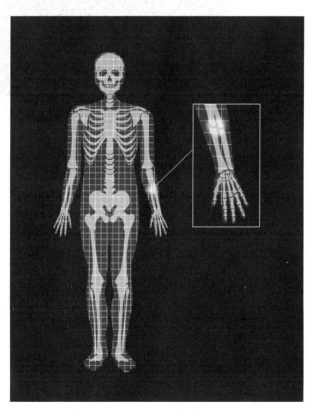

12. Hologram of skeletal structure
on black background

When I am looking at someone's aura, I always see that on a black background, when working at distance, anyway. The aura will show up as white all around the hologram, and if there is a hole in the aura anywhere, I will look at that particular area and smooth the energy back out, creating a harmonious flow.

Some people see colours around a body, and sometimes I do too. Not all that often however. People will say different coloured auras mean different things. For me, I don't see colours very often and it doesn't affect my work in the slightest. If you are unable to see colours around a body, don't worry. The aura is what is important. If you can't see it you will definitely be able to feel it. To try and see it look slightly to the right or left, off of the client you are facilitating the healing of. Let your gaze be loose and allow the aura to come into your field of awareness/sight.

You want the human being in question to have a glowing, full aura as in the following picture.

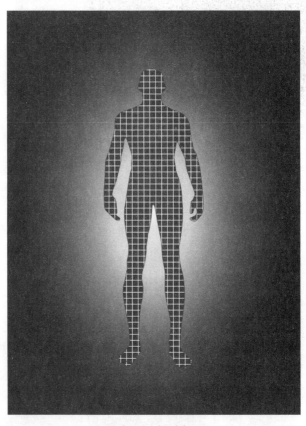

13. A glowing healthy aura

Energy Cords

A lot of people have energy cords within their energetic framework. In the picture below I have shown them on a black background but that is not how I see them. I don't see them on any particular background. This picture is purely for illustration purposes.

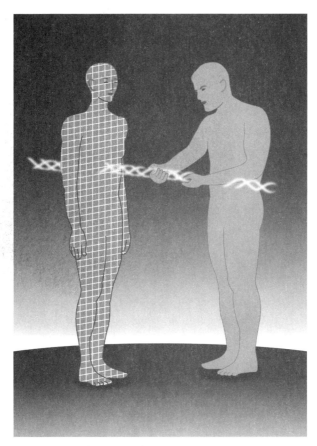

14. Hologram with energy cord coming out

I will run my hands over someone's body, and my hands will vibrate. When I feel my hands vibrate I know there is stuck energy, in the form of an energy cord, within the field of this human being. I will feel it, and then see it. I will grab it like a piece of rope. When you are aware, even if this is being done at distance, you will feel something being pulled from your body. I do this in my seminars and workshops and the results can be instantaneous. Remove the cord and the energy can flow freely.

As I pull the energy out from the body I see it turning into light, brilliant white light. Some people get concerned that this energy will affect them. Remember your intention is everything. Know that it will not affect you and it won't. See it turn into light and fizzle back out into the ether, to be used for good wherever needed, and that will be so. You are the master of your mind, the controller of your soul. You must know this. Intention is everything.

Once I have removed an energy cord, the body can self-heal, as the energy can flow freely. The patterns of light within the hologram simply re-organize themselves. I don't know how or why, they just do. I see so many people just wanting to pump energy into the client that they are healing and the effort is wasted. Why? Because you are not eliminating the stuck energy.

Remove the energy cord first then the healing takes place. We are not running energy though our bodies when using Star Magic. We are using light and the information contained within the light to facilitate healing. We are simply re-arranging patterns and transferring or exchanging information.

Once the energy cord has been removed, it often leaves a hole in the energy field, so I will then fill that back up with light. I don't actually fill it back up: I watch it fill back up. Once it is full it stops. This you can see, probably with your mind's eye at first, and then with practise, it's like you are looking through your physical eyes.

During the facilitation of healing sessions, I have become aware of the movement of energy, in that it tends to move in waves. When a hologram is flowing perfectly, like waves rolling into the seashore, I know that the human being is healthy, as the energy is flowing smoothly. When there is an issue of any kind, I will see an adverse pattern in the wave flow, and so, to correct it, all I need to do is run an inverse wave pattern. In other words, manipulate the energy flow in the opposite direction, thus causing the wave patterns to start flowing back towards the seashore, in a rhythmic and seamless fashion, with no interruptions.

It may seem from reading this and viewing these diagrams that I am suggesting you view holograms in this way too. Nothing could be further from the truth. I am simply offering my perspective. We all see differently. You will need to drop into the healing zone and feel your own way. There is no right or wrong. There is simply your way and my way. And maybe our ways will be the same. Maybe they will be similar. Maybe they won't.

Zero-Point or Inverted Field

When I feel or see the issue within the hologram I will place my hands on the hologram in two locations. Those locations can be anywhere, not necessarily near a particular dis-ease or injury. I will feel drawn to two particular places. There is a pulling sensation. Once both hands are in place I enter what is referred to as the zero-point field. I don't know why it's called that. I have read a few books on physics and quantum mechanics but most of the information doesn't stack up for me. It doesn't feel right.

I actually feel there is an inverted field and this is where the magic happens. If you look at a swan gliding gracefully on the water it looks as though it is moving with zero effort. Yet, underneath the water it is paddling with its feet. Now the feet are not level with the water, they are underneath. The water level would be the zero-point field. Nothing is actually happening there, not in the case of the swan anyway.

It's underneath the water, in the inverted field where the magic is happening to make the swan move across the water. I am no scientist but I know what I know and what I see every day when I am facilitating healings and I know there is an inverted field that runs deep within, into the space that is all around us and is us.

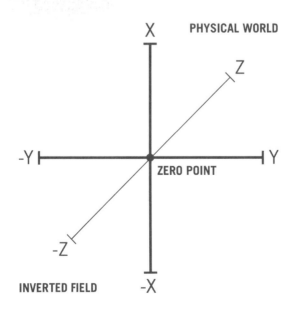

15. The Inverted Field

The diagram on the previous page shows a graph. You may have seen a graph like this at school. The lines x, y and z represent everything that is happening in the physical world. 0 represents the zero-point field where everything is said to be created from. Lines – x, – y and – z represent the inverted field that extends way down deep, into infinity. This is where the real magic happens. This is un-ventured territory for most people.

I am suggesting that you go there and explore. You will be amazed. Cup your hand and hold it out in front of you right now. Look at the space in your hand. That space in your hand reaches to infinite depths. Imagine the fingernail on your little finger. If you could shrink down 100 times smaller than it you could walk through the nail and into a whole new world.

Well, the inverted field is like that. This physical world is 0.00000000000 000000000000000000001% of the truth. There is probably a lot more zeros than that. I am just trying to make a point. The swan on the water represents the physical world. Imagine that the swan was swimming on a lake the size of the moon. The huge moon-sized lake below the water level is where the truth lies, and remember that the moon is limited. It's only a certain size. The infinite depths of the inverted field are just that, infinite.

Why do scientists refer to it as the zero-point field? Maybe it's because they want us to stop looking? Maybe it's because they themselves haven't really got a clue what is going on?

If a man were to punch another man then you may say this all took place in between +x and +y, in the physical world. But did it? Yes, he may have punched the other man but what about the thought that triggered the punch? Or maybe the thought that triggered the emotion that triggered the punch? And what triggered the thought? Maybe an emotion triggered the thought. If so, what triggered the emotion? It was invisible. Somewhere between -x and -y, in the inverted field.

If I were to hold a quartz crystal the size of a one-penny coin (similar to the thumb nail) in front of me and then crawl inside of it and venture off to Mars, or to Egypt when Nefertiti was alive, would I be going any distance to do this if it all took place inside the crystal?

Maybe there is no inverted field? Maybe there is no zero-point? Maybe you can fold space in half? Maybe you can bend space and by bending it you can open it up to infinite depths? If this is the case, then there must be an inverted field. Or is there?

The field becomes inverted upon entry and before entry it is the zero-point. It is actually both but then again both are just labels, which in real time, do not describe anything. Whatever takes place between +x and +y and -x and -y are all one stream of consciousness. Zero separation. Nothing is isolated. For it to be isolated the space between -x and -y would have to be separate from the space between +x and +y. That would mean the man literally just punched the other man, and that, my friend, is impossible. No action can ever be taken without a trigger, an impulse and firing of neurons from within the nervous system, activated by consciousness, the invisible controller that no scientist has ever detected.

> **Here is a simple exercise for you to do now:**
> Close your eyes and drop into your heart space. Then open your heart like a doorway or a Star Gate. Walk to the edge of this Star Gate and look out. This is the Universal Database, contained in the inverted field. The Star Gate is the zero-point, if you feel they are separate. Maybe they are both the inverted field or both the zero-point.
>
> Either way this Star Gate is your entrance to the live streams of never ending information. You must make love to this space and it will make love back to you. Bond here. Enjoy it here. Be comfortable here and let the magic unfold.

When people embark on this spiritual journey and they start to see the light and feel the vibration of love they think or feel maybe, that they are on the homeward stretch.

Nothing could be further from the truth. This is where the journey gets started. Light comes from dark. The Universe was birthed from empty space, the inverted field. Light comes from black holes. True light is darkness. Here lies the key to darkness. And darkness is not bad or evil, it's perfection in its truest nature. There is no separation between the physical and the non-physical world, the physical and the inverted field.

Light and dark are one and to truly flourish in this human life you must invite your shadow self, the darker aspect of you to the surface, the aspect of you that lurks within the inverted field. That is the inverted field. It must be invited to the surface to be loved and nurtured and in doing so set free. And once you set it free you will realize that it was always free. An aspect of your own soul that had lowered its vibration was always a part of your wholeness and has now raised its vibration in line with the rest of the whole.

This is what Star Magic brings. A dominant love that is both masculine and feminine. Not just airy-fairy human love, based on misunderstanding and softness. Spirit/source isn't soft. It's both kind and harsh in its purest and rawest form. Human kind is now moving into a phase to assimilate this. You, at your core are a black hole. The light comes from the black hole. Star Magic will take you beyond light.

Some people are not ready. If you are reading this book, then you most definitely are. The truth isn't all sunshine and rainbows. The truth, in its rawest form is harsh. Love is intense. The purest love that pours from the central abyss is too powerful for most. When you play with Star Magic you will know this and experience it first-hand. Your shadow self cannot hide within the inverted field when you utilize Star Magic.

The fearful stay in light where they are comfortable. Light is human love. Dark is God. Dark is Jesus. Dark is you and me at the core of our being and dark is the new light, the essence of who and what we truly are.

3D stuff/baggage/drama is the outer shell. Beyond this there is light and beyond light there is darkness, empty space. Once the illusion drops we see light and think we are home but we are not. We must go beyond light, to nothing. This is the inverted field. To transform humanity, we must unleash the innermost demons, which are not really demons. They are beautiful aspects of the one stream of consciousness. The dark foundation that gave birth to light.

When you start to play with Star Magic the truth will be revealed. Star Magic works, easily, it's teachable or sharable and that is all that matters to me. Trust me – if I can do it you can too.

Once you feel the two locations on the hologram you let nature take its course. Your job is to observe and use your imagination to produce results. Be aware of what you notice and follow your instincts.

ᚲ

I had someone whose hearing had suddenly gone, in her left ear, and she was constantly off balance. As soon as I dropped into the healing zone I saw, in another reality this same lady in a swimming pool of light. The light poured into her ear and I saw, in the ear that couldn't hear, a rubber bung or stopper. I imagined the light pushing this stopper out from her ear.

As soon as it did we switched immediately to another reality where she was on a tight rope. She was wobbling. I used my imagination to widen the rope. I then made it hard and it turned into a wide plank of wood. The lady stopped wobbling and I came back into the room, popped out of my healing zone and was back in the third-dimensional world of form.

Months later she contacted me and told me everything was still as good as it was after the healing session. Does this make logical sense? No. Does it work? Yes. Why? Because imagination infused with a loving and knowing intention, mixed with information (light) is "more real" than the pages in this book. The pages in this book are everything but real.

By feeling the two points on the body or in the energy field of the person you are healing you get access to the information that can heal her/him just like above. Something else that works very well is to find two points on the body or in the energy field and create an imaginary line or wave of light between the two points. It can be like a laser beam of light or energy. Once you have created the laser beam with your imagination (which is reality) you then know that this laser beam represents a pattern that is causing an injury/illness or dysfunctional situation, that once broken will create an environment whereby the healing can take place.

What you are doing is collapsing a wave that no longer serves this human being. You are entangling the wave or energy/light with the issue that needs to be resolved and once you collapse it, the issue or ailment disappears along with the wave of light. Just simply see it blow up or disappear.

Group Healing

In my workshops I always do a group healing regardless of how many people there are. The more the merrier. The more people there are in a room, the more energy and light we have to play with. It's super powerful. I have been in groups where our energy has blown the power out, in the houses, and in the surrounding area of our energy-healing workshop. The power tends to blow out everywhere apart from the room that we are in. It always makes me smile. Alarms ring first on cars, houses, office buildings, all at once, so you know the power surge coming from our room has caused it. Love!

When I facilitate a group healing I will join everyone's energy field together and then bring up a holographic group blueprint or master hologram. I will work on the blueprint and then the healing filters down into everyone in the room. As above, so below. Inside this hologram I can see a multitude of different ailments but to focus on them all is too much. So I blast intense light throughout the entire hologram and this normally does the trick. For even better results bring your master group hologram up in space inside an inverted pyramid. See this spinning clockwise. This inverted pyramid will be inside a sphere that is spinning anti-clockwise. Visualize this. It is extremely powerful and enhances the experience.

I work in exactly the same way that I do in a private healing, and it is very effective. Remember the light/energy knows what is best, and my intention is everything. In these group situations I tend to trance out. I used to think that I knew what was happening, precisely, and it wasn't until a friend of mine said, "*Jerry, are you aware of everything that is happening?*" I said yes, thinking that I was, but it wasn't until she explained what my own body was doing that I thought, well actually, maybe I am not as in control as I thought I was. It's like I am taken over. So I recorded the next workshop so I could see myself afterwards – very strange.

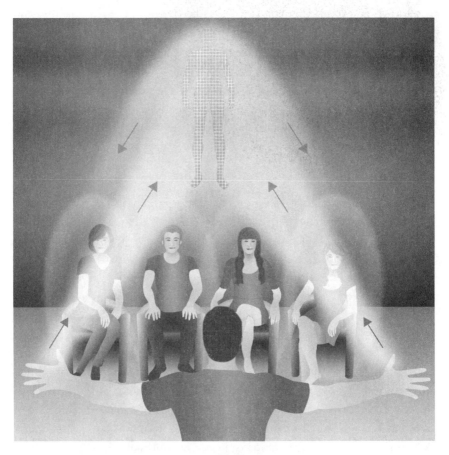

16. Audience with hologram above,
with Jerry blasting energy into it

People will say to me that they looked up during the healing and I wasn't there, or they saw an Egyptian man stood where I was supposed to be, or a man with black skin. It's really interesting. What happens during these healings is all of my multi-dimensional selves, come back home, into me, to this space to help me facilitate the healing. So when people don't see me but another man, woman or being, they are just seeing another aspect of me.

It's totally normal. For some it may seem a little freaky, if you're not used to it. I have recorded one or two group healings but now I tend not to. They are so personal and intimate, and I take people on such deep journeys, that what arises can be often upsetting when people are facing their fears, and releasing deep seated emotions from this lifetime, or previous/parallel ones. Past lives only really exist in our mind, when we think of linear time.

Really, every life is happening now. All lives everywhere are unfolding now within the field – just in another space, on another vibration.

There really only ever is now.

16

Basic Healing Ways and Visualizations

I am going to share with you a variety of ways, some more basic, others more advanced and a selection of intermediary ways to bridge the gap between the two, in this book. Really and truthfully they are all easy. I have just found it is easier to remember when the information is offered in this way. I will share ways that you can use to facilitate the healing of others and ways that you can use to facilitate your own healing.

These ways come in the form of visualizations. Remember your imagination is reality. There are so many creative ways to create health by changing the pattern of a dis-ease, injury or illness as well as enhance business performance and relationships.

These following visualizations are all very basic ways and you can practise with them straight away. They will get you into the right space, so you can start to use your imagination and intention in a simple fashion. You may have seen some of them before. I wanted to include them because if you haven't or even if you have, you need to lay the foundation, before stepping across (not up) to the next level or space.

It will set you up perfectly to use the more advanced ways, which are not really advanced. I say they are advanced as they require a little more letting go. Please practise with the basic ways first before going onto the more advanced options, later in the book. It will build your confidence.

Before we commence it's important that you have an idea of what the human body looks like internally. It's no good a client saying to you that they have cancer of the spleen and you don't have a clue what the spleen is or where it's located. I am not a doctor, physician and have never studied the human body. Often, when people came to me, at first I didn't have a clue what the medical term meant, or where that part of the body was. So I looked it up. It's not a necessity with the more advanced ways as you by-pass everything logical, and it's more effective. But to start with, get to know the body. It will give you that basic knowledge, which will elevate your levels of confidence. On the following page you find some inside views of the human body.

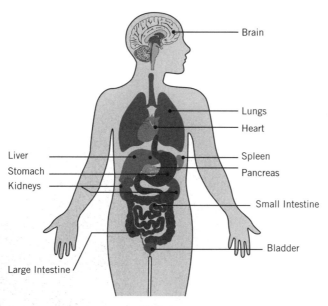

17. Organs

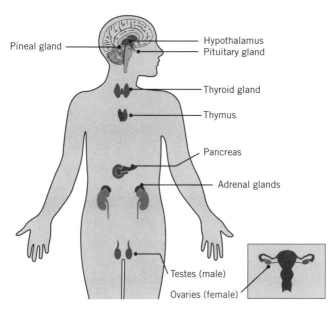

18. Endocrine system

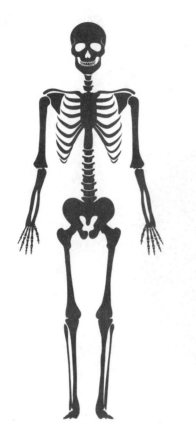

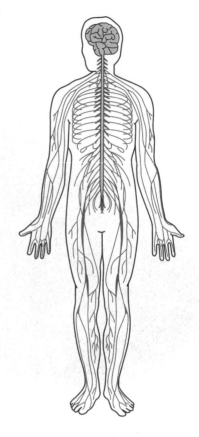

19. Skeletal structure   20. Nervous system

It is important to know that when you are utilizing all of the following visualizations that you keep your hands on the hologram to feel when the ailment has subsided. For example, if someone has a stiff shoulder and I run my hands over their hologram and feel the two places on their body, where my hands are drawn to, it will feel tingly, stiff, stuck or some sensation that you feel or see is not right. Sometimes by simply acknowledging that this area needs to be sorted the light re-arranges itself and it just happens. Not always though. And when it doesn't you can use your imagination until it does. Once you remember how to feel and see what floats into your consciousness you can use it until the feelings on your hands subside. The stuckness or magnetic pull or the tingly feeling will simply disappear and you know that there has been a shift. Sometimes it will show up in the physical body instantaneously and other times it filters in over days or weeks, sometimes longer.

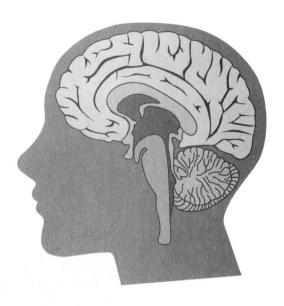

21. Brain

The following visualizations can be effective. None of them are set in stone. All I am trying to demonstrate is how you can utilize your imagination and play around with creative ways in the quantum field to create change in the physical reality of someone you are facilitating the healing of. Remember the observer affects the observed. When your intention and knowing is powerful enough you will create miracles.

Explosions of Love

There are no diagrams in this next section because I want you to use your imagination. Start playing and visualizing and putting your own spin on things.

OK. First, Imagine the human being's body or hologram you are facilitating the healing of. Let's say they have a tumour. You can imagine packing the inside of their body with sticks or blocks of dynamite. This dynamite is created by love. You pack the sticks or blocks (which I see in the shape of hearts) into the body, all around the area that needs healing. Once that is packed out I will spread a few random pieces of dynamite throughout the body. Then with my imaginary detonator, I will blow them up, and then I see an explosion of white light.

97

The entire body turns to light and totally disappears. It's important that you don't combat the tumour. To do so would enhance its strength. What you are doing is creating a different reality. I have cleared many tumours with this method – it works. The more intense the explosion and the more vivid it is in your imagination, the more real it becomes. You will see, after using this way that imagination really is reality. Do not use force with this method. Use love.

After the first explosion, if you can still see some of the tumour left, go again. I have had sessions whereby the tumour has cleared with one explosion. Other times it's taken several healing sessions using the same way. I will combine this with the Split Body Way I share in the chapter "Cellular Level", which is an advanced way. These two, combined, work wonders. The explosions of love eliminate the symptoms, and sometimes the cause, but the Split Body Way will always eliminate the cause. Together they are very powerful.

Injections

Injections of light are easy to administer and are great for any aches, pains, injuries. They work with broken bones, swellings of any kind, knees, elbows or shoulder strains. They are great with fibromyalgia. If you use this way with fibromyalgia you may want to use the Split Body Way too.

These are so simple. You visualize a syringe, full of light, and inject it into the person's body. If your client has an area that needs attention, you will probably see this as stagnant black energy or it may show up as a colour for you that is different from the rest of the body. Simply inject the white light, into that area, and see it transform the body back into alignment with the rest of the energy.

As you begin to use Star Magic more and more, you will start to see the body as I do. You will see it as a vibrating mass of energy. This is the next level of Star Magic, and once you move across to this level, facilitating a healing is even easier. Once you open up to that stage, a number of these visualizations will be unnecessary, but for now, please use them.

Freeze and Explode

This way is great for everything. Simply locate the area that needs attention. Visualize it filling up with water (the water is light/energy) and then freezing. Then with your intention, see the ice explode, and in its place remains beautiful crystal white light.

Freeze and Melt

This way is the same as the last. However instead of exploding, the ice melts, carrying away the negative or stuck energy. You see it run from the body.

Pacman Approach

Do you remember the video game Pacman? All of those little round things with large mouths, racing around eating everything in sight? Well this way resembles something similar. If you have a client with a cyst or cancerous tumour, it's perfect. You can locate the symptoms of the dis-ease (the growth), and then see all of these little Pac men, like white blood cells, surrounding the tumour or cyst, and literally see them eating it away. It sounds bizarre but they actually do work, and very well. You can literally see the tumour disappearing before your very eyes.

Here, you are in a way, combatting the tumour but I don't see it like this. I will visualize the tumour as a food source for the little Pac men. So in my reality I am doing them a kind deed by feeding them. Your intention is everything. Use it wisely. Let go and play, my friend.

Flames

Flames work well for healing. If I am facilitating a healing, the client often feels hot or cold. This is the healing taking place. So in our healing practise, when using Star Magic, it is imperative that we use heat and cold to our advantage. I always use purple or electric blue flames, although sometimes the flames will show up in a different colour. If that is the case, just go with it. The energy/light knows what is best. Be flexible. A rigid mind is a destructive mind.

I use flames to cleanse a client. I will see the human being engulfed in flames, from head to toe and hold them in that space for a few minutes. I also use flames inside the body, to bring swelling down, and also to burn away any stagnant build-ups of unwanted energy. Flames are powerful and can transmute negative emotions too. All of these ways are powerful, with the right intention. I allow a variety of different colours into my space if that is what is available to use. Violet or electric blue work the best.

Waterfall

I also use a waterfall of liquid light to cleanse my clients. I visualize them stood, or lying under a waterfall and liquid light is raining down on them, cleansing their body and mind and moving any unwanted energy on. I see this liquid light fill up the entire inside of their body and the body becomes pure brilliant white light. The body becomes the waterfall and everything else that no longer serves the human being in question, runs away.

Marble Body

This basic way is one of my favourites. Visualize the inside of the body filling up with marbles. See the entire body full of them, with no space in between. Imagine if you picked that body up it would make a clunking sound if you shook it, with all those little marbles stacked up against each other. Once you have visualized the body full of marbles, see the inside of the marbles glowing brightly. Next turn up the light. See them become brighter and brighter. Once they are as bright as you can make them, count from five back to zero, and watch them explode, all at once, blasting any stuck energy from the body, and leaving a space of brilliant white light.

Lightning

This is great for the nervous system or anything neurological. It is perfect also for stimulating limbs that may have suffered in an accident. Simply see lightning crackling down from the sky. See it hitting the top of the human being's head, and start to stimulate the nervous system. See the energy travel down through the brain, down the spine, along the arms and legs until the entire nervous system is glowing. If you have reached the level of seeing the nervous system, in the colours I have mentioned earlier, you will see it turn from red to green. If you can't it will still work.

Fireworks

These are great for clearing a busy mind. You can see thoughts racing around inside your client's head and simply visualize each thought as a firework shooting, igniting, and exploding into beautiful colours and shapes, and leaving behind a trail of emptiness. The mind after all can be very destructive, and when our ego is in control and running riot, this can be a great way to bridge the gap between noise and stillness of the mind. As the thoughts, which are light, explode, you can visualize an electrical charge of clean energy pulsating through the nervous system and throughout the body, cleansing, nourishing and filling it full of harmonious and intelligent power as it does.

All of these ways are created by your imagination. Let go and try them. Let go a little further and see what else flows into your consciousness. Let go and the light and energy will take on a life of its own, until you become an observer of the imagination.

17

Intermediate Healing Ways

The next three ways I will share with you require a little more insight/ letting go, a greater ability to see with your mind's eye and a greater awareness, to feel the vibrational light/energy position, of an illness or dis-ease. These ways are also very good for simply clearing and cleansing the energy system of anyone who asks you to facilitate their healing, in general terms. For example, if they want a general service, as I sometimes call it. Just like we take a car to the garage to be serviced, it's great to have a Star Magic cleansing session to clean, clear and balance the energy centres and smooth over the energy field through the holographic blueprint.

Light Hands

I call this way, Light Hands, because you are using your hands as a tool. You will need to scan the blueprint of the body you are about to work on and either see or feel where the stagnant energy build-up is. Once you locate the area, you place your hands inside the human being's body, and see your hands completely turn to light. Most of the time my hands turn into a bright white light, but there have been times when they glow pink, green, blue, silver and other colours. Be flexible and go with the light/ energy colour. It doesn't have to make logical sense. *Remember Star Magic is rooted in love, not in logic.*

If it's a simple energy blockage I will bring light in through my crown chakra, fire up my nervous system, and see light and information, in the form of codes, race down my arms and power up my hands. I will keep this strong flow the entire time with my intention. The light emanating from my hands will get stronger and stronger and light up the area of the body I am working on, sometimes the entire body. Clients will tell me they can feel something inside of them. Others will say, *"Jerry, I felt your hands inside my body."* Remember to keep the flow of light, energy and information inside your body cool. See the image on the following page (and also the color insert).

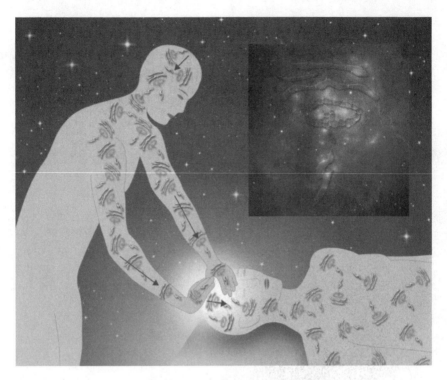

22. Codes flowing through the healer's body and hands via
the crown chakra into the client's body

The codes you see coming through my body are what sets Star Magic apart from any other healing modality. These codes are what I downloaded on my trip to Alpha Centuri. If you come to one of my workshops I will align you with this extra-terrestrial frequency. If you meditate on this book you hold in your hands, it's possible for the same alignment to take place. You will know when you have triggered this set of light codes because everything will shift. It's an experience like no other.

If there is an energy blockage I will place my hands around its supposed location, and light up my hands using exactly the same method. I will shine such an intense light on the area the blockage (which could have taken on the physical manifestation of a growth) is supposed to be, and at the same time see no growth. Remember I am here not to battle the growth or the stagnant energy. The growth doesn't exist in my world. The light I am, changes the patterns of light within the human being's holographic blueprint.

In times like these it's great to know your way around the body, so having a basic understanding of where things are is important. I also want to point out that if you don't know your way around the body it will not stop the facilitation of the healing. Know that the light will change what is necessary. Someone could have a dis-ease in their liver and you could place your hands on their head, or away from their head in space. The outcome will still be the same. *Knowing* is the golden key. Believing is the anchor that will hold you back.

Chakra Release

Again, you will need to be able to feel or see, or maybe both, the energy centres known as chakras, in the body. Most people know the basic seven.

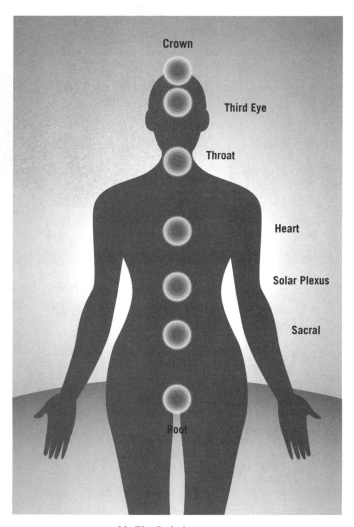

23. The 7-chakra-system

I also work with 2 different 13-chakra-systems. It's important to note that you must choose which system to work with. The basic 7-chakra-system is great for working through issues, here and now, within the physical and emotional bodies. The same goes for the 13-in-body chakra-system. This, however, is also important to use when activating the higher levels of your spiritual capabilities.

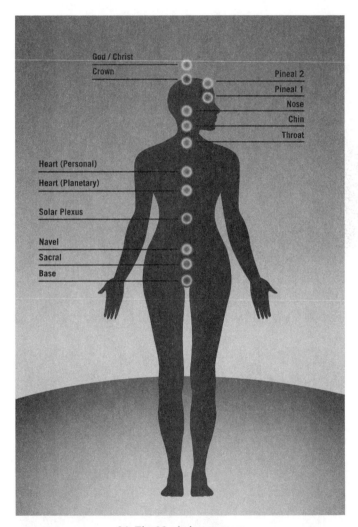

God / Christ
Crown
Pineal 2
Pineal 1
Nose
Chin
Throat
Heart (Personal)
Heart (Planetary)
Solar Plexus
Navel
Sacral
Base

24. The 13-chakra-system

Here is a picture of the 13 body chakras that the Egyptians used. The space between each one is approximately 7. 2 cm or the distance from your thumb to your little finger. You can place one hand next to the other moving all of

104

the way up your body (from your Perineum to your Crown Chakra) and you will hit each one. Perfect geometry. Coincidence?

The reason I use it is because this is what the Egyptians used, and when I was being shown how to facilitate the healing of others inside the Ancient Mystery Schools, this was prominent. It's closely linked with sacred geometry and so the whole YOU-Niverse.

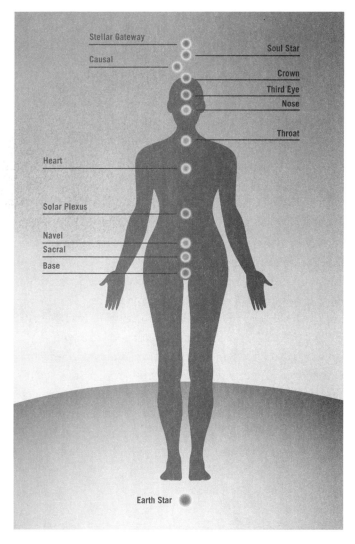

25. The 13 fifth-dimensional-chakra-system
(in and out of body)

It's important to anchor yourself into the fifth-dimensional light frequencies ready for ascension, through the Star Systems. We will discuss this later on in the book, however I wanted to make you aware of it now.

I want to point something very important out to you at this stage. The Causal, Soul Star, Stella Gateway and Christ Self chakras are not really chakras. They have been referred to as chakras by others for many years and I understand why. People can see or feel something there, or they simply know something is there, but they have not tuned into them fully to know exactly what is happening.

These four points should really be called Transmission Centres. They make up a very important part of our fifth-dimensional spiritual nervous system, that connects us to fifth-dimensional light. There is a tube of light that runs from many meters below our physical body to many metres above it. This tube runs between the in- and out-point of our fifth-dimensional activation chamber, an integral element of the ascension process. The activation chamber is a part of our fifth-dimensional extra-terrestrial light body. Yes, you have one too. We all do. We are all Star Seeds.

In this book I am not going into the full detail of this light body. It's not necessary for you to heal. I felt it very important, however, to mention this for clarity. There are a lot of people sharing information on this particular chakra topic. While it is great that people are being made aware of something else it can be a little misleading at the same time. Know that these points exist and that they are Transmission Centres, not chakras.

It is important for our main seven or thirteen (in body) chakras to stay open, aligned and fluid to optimize our health and wellbeing. The Transmission Centres, however, are simply there to allow the flow of information from other star systems and our own matrix of human potential, including every other reality being lived holographically, in the now. In my next book I am going to go into this topic in detail as its very important.

Back to the 7-chakra-system; our chakras in our body are like ice-cream cones, for most people. Large at one end, and smaller at the other. It's like having the two small points meeting in the middle of the body, and the larger end of the ice-cream cone on the outside.

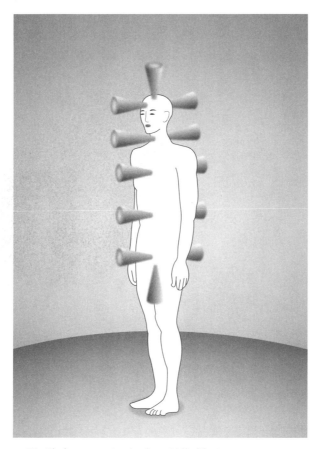

26. Chakras meeting in the middle like ice cream cones

Now when your chakras are like this, which most people's are, much emotion is carried/stuck, in the smaller end. Stuff gets blocked. What Star Magic enables you to do is open those chakras fully so that they become free flowing cylinders, straight through the body. This releases you from the game of duality. Use the 7-chakra-system for this.

Step one is to open each chakra to its full capacity and step two is to clean the inside of each chakra. Step three is to merge these chakras into one unified field. Now, not everyone is ready for this, so you are going to need your awareness. The great thing is that the client's inner self will not allow this to happen if they are not ready. You can communicate with their spirit or inner self and ask, *"Is John or Sarah ready for me to do this?"* You will need to listen carefully. The voice that will answer is often softly spoken, and easy to miss.

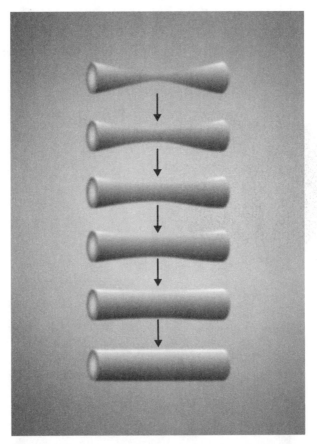

27. Chakras transitioning into cylinders through clearing

You may think it's your so-called imagination, and so you must learn to feel and trust. Communicating with spirit and opening the lines of dialogue, is a must for you. You may feel the answer rather than hear it. Maybe both. Or you will just know. However it happens for you – allow it.

Step One

To open each chakra you will need mental strength as you will come up against resistance. More so in certain cases, depending on who you are working with. Opening the chakras can also bring up deep-seated emotions, which have been clogged inside the energy centres for a long time. To open these chakras you simply visualize the smaller end of the cone becoming larger, until it's the same width as the wide end. You do that on both sides of the body until you have created a cylinder.

You are going to need your Third Eye for this and I am going to share with you some tips and strategies later in the book, so you can open your Third Eye and start to utilize it fully. Creating the cylinder cannot be forced, however a little gentle persuasion is sometimes necessary.

Step Two

Once the cylinder has been created and there is a channel from one side of the body to the other, any stuck energy can be moved in a much easier fashion.

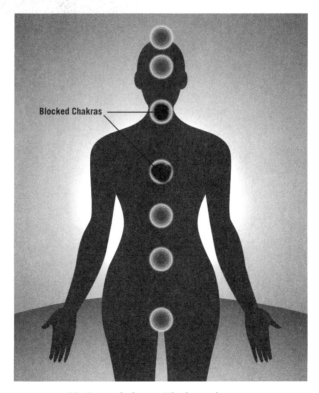

28. Open chakras with clogged energy

You will notice energy inside, sometimes; stuck energy that doesn't need to be there, karmic residue that has been there for many years. Three ways to move this energy on are as follows.

1. Shine light through from one end to the other and watch it filter through. It's not always as easy as this because the old stuff doesn't want to shift.
2. So you can adopt this way of clearing the chakras. Imagine the cylinder is like a straw. A large one at that, but you could shrink it in your mind if it helps. Put your lips/mouth around the end of the cylinder and blow extremely hard and see this stuck energy moving on until the pathway is clear for you, and the clean energy can flow freely.
3. Sometimes I see big chunks of energy. They look like clumps of coal or rock. They are very heavy and don't want to budge. If this is the case I will take an imaginary rod of light and push it through the chakra. On occasions it takes a lot of mental strength, but I will not stop until I have pushed that rod of light all the way through, and have seen the clump of coal or rock, fly out of the other side. Remember to see that stuck, blocked up energy turn to white light upon its release. The size of the rod that you will use is just small enough to fit inside of the chakra, so no stuck energy escapes being pushed out.

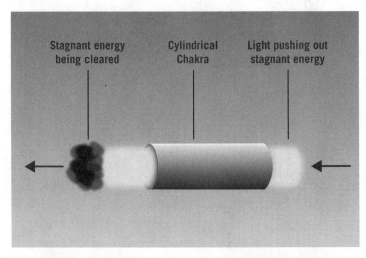

29. Blocked chakra – light pushing out stagnant energy

Infinity Sign

30. Infinity sign

The above picture is the infinity sign. It resembles the consistent flow of life. I was shown how to run this through the body once you have cleaned and balanced the chakras.

Again you can use your mind or you may find it easier to run this through the body with your hand. Simply see the holographic blueprint in front of you. Start at the head and move out to the right of the body, then bring it back in through the right hip, and out of the other side of the body, and down through the feet, creating an S shape. You then continue on and mirror the shape on the other side, creating a figure of eight or the Infinity Sign.

You must repeat this eleven times creating perfect flow. This resembles all life and all things in the YOU-Niverse, flowing as one complete and whole energy source. This includes the human being you are facilitating the healing of. I questioned this at first. I was speaking to my guides and saying, *"But we are divine intelligence. We are all connected anyway."* They just kept telling me to use it. So I conducted my own experiment.

I got twelve human beings that all had a little something that needed to be healed. My plan was to use Star Magic every day until the client was healed. Six people I used the Infinity Sign on and six I didn't. Call it coincidence or not but the humans that I used the Infinity Sign on were healed within a day, some two. The ones I didn't use the Infinity Sign on took longer.

So Star Magic is powerful with or without the Infinity sign but if it helps heal faster, then use it. It certainly does something and this is a perfect example of working with light. It doesn't have to make sense. It's rooted in love, not in logic. It's knowing versus believing. Let go and allow things to take place. You may come up with a whole bunch of other ways to use the light. If you do, then use it. Do what works for you.

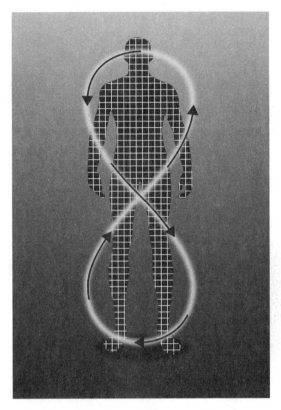

31. Energy flowing through the body in
the shape of the infinity symbol

Stars, Love & Earth

This way is great for yourself and others. Bring up the holographic blueprint of the other human being, or yourself. See it in front of you. Move into their space and open your heart chakra. See the light pouring from your heart into theirs, through the back of the hologram. So it is like you are stood or sat behind their hologram. You then bring Earth light/energy up from the ground and into their feet, see it travel up through the body until it connects with the light from your heart. Then bring light down from the stars.

See it penetrate the top of their crown and move down until it meets the Earth and heart energies/lights. When the three combine, mixed with a super-focused intention, sprinkled with the imagination of both the healer and the client (yes get them involved if you wish), you will bring about rapid healing. Play with the light. Play with the information.

Sometimes I will see geometry flowing through the light – the flower of life, Metatron's Cube, Tree of Life and more basic shapes such as squares, triangles and cubes. Remember these shapes contain information. They are intelligent. Other more complex shapes such as the Christ Consciousness Grid will move into my space and take on a life of its own along with the mission-critical Star Magic Light Codes. Notice what happens. Observe. Let the light flow and watch the magic take pace. Tune in and experience.

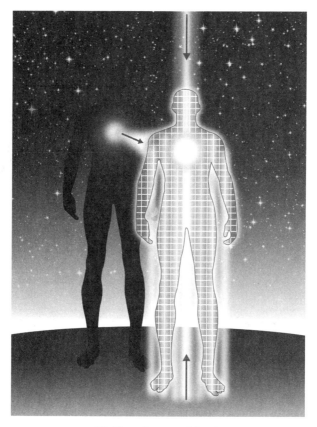

32. Stars, Love, and Earth

Co-Creating As You Go

All of the above ways work and are open to be changed. I am simply giving you some ideas of what has worked for me. Now, I want to share with you what happens when you let your mind go and it flows freely on its own. This for me is when the real miracles happen.

I had a lady who came to see me at a spiritual festival. I often do fifteen-minute demonstrations at a festival. This lady sat down with a painful shoulder and her spine was bent and leaning to one side. Her relationships with men had been traumatic throughout her life. It is no wonder that all of her pain seemed to be on the right hand side of her body. The right hand side is male. The left is female. It is opposite when it comes to the brain so remember this.

She sat down in her chair and I was drawn to her stomach area. I placed one hand in her energy field in front of her stomach and one hand in the energy field on the right hand side of her body, pointing towards her shoulder. Very rarely do I touch anyone. As soon as I did this I saw a green bolt of light move from her base chakra, up through her spine. It shot up and out of her head. It did this three times and as it did her spine straightened up. A few minutes later she burst out crying. Once she stood up her shoulder felt much better. It wasn't totally gone but it was relieved in a major way.

The next day she contacted me and said that she could stand up straight now and her shoulder was completely better. She said what was really interesting and amazing though, was the fact that her relationship with a certain man in her life has completely changed. It happened overnight. He was acting differently. Everything seemed like the way it should be. Whatever was causing her pain was some emotional issue towards men. The information contained within the light changed this. Once it released, the physical healing took place also.

A lady contacted me with stomach problems, migraines, low energy, skin disorders and a few other symptoms. She had had a miscarriage, and lost her husband. She said the last few years of her life had been a real struggle.

I dropped into my healing zone and entered her space. I saw her as a little girl. She wasn't happy. I could also see the inner resistance within their own relationship, the woman and her inner child that is. I know this because I asked them – in another reality by introducing them – to give each other a cuddle. They wouldn't. I could see some black energy in between them. I didn't know what it meant but knew it shouldn't be there.

I opened my heart chakra fully, shone light over the dark area until it was consumed by the light. As soon as I did this they moved towards each other and started cuddling. Next I saw a silver fish appear in my own hand. What is this I asked my guides? They told me to put this fish inside of her body, so I did.

Once inside her body the fish turned into a silver light and started swimming around her body. It consumed her entire inside. Seconds later a Unicorn burst through my own chest, swooped down and they drifted onto the

Unicorn's back. The Unicorn then took them through space to the healing Pools of Consciousness in Egypt (we will discuss these soon) and put them down. A being then came and carried them off the Unicorn's back and laid them in the healing pools. They cuddled and played in the energy until they became one.

Moments later the lady was lying back down on her bed and her inner child was fully submerged into her. They had fully reconnected on the deepest possible level. Within days the lady felt so much better. We did one more healing two weeks later and she has had no issues since. How can the removal of an invisible black energy, a silver fish, a mythical Unicorn, an Egyptian Being and an imaginary healing pool create such significant healing in the physical world?

I knew a gentleman who was told he needed a knee operation and that there was no other way of him gaining his ability to walk properly without it. This may sound a little crazy (not that Unicorns and silver fish don't) but it's so simple and yet it created a miracle.

This gentleman was in his fifties, a keen tennis player and hadn't played for over a year. He was waiting on knee surgery but felt there was another option. I visualized his hologram and Usain Bolt appeared in my space. I instantly thought, what if this guy had Usain Bolt's legs; he would be playing tennis better than ever. So I removed one leg and fitted a version of Usain Bolt's left leg. I then thought, this guy is fifty-three. It would be great if he had two new, younger and fresher legs. So I removed his right leg too and put another Usain Bolt leg in its place. I saw this guy running and playing tennis like he did when he was in his prime.

After the healing session he told me he felt good. He played tennis the very same afternoon. What was incredible to me was this. The next week he contacted me and said, *"Jerry, you know it's very strange but my left leg feels better too. I didn't tell you but I had a nasty niggle in that leg. I didn't tell you as I could still function but now it feels as good as the other one too."*

So you see, let your imagination flow. It doesn't have to make sense. Drop into the zone and run with whatever is in front of you. Flow and co-create alternate realities and quantum entangle the two.

18

Crystals and Geometry

Crystals themselves are divine beings. They carry within them intelligence. You can communicate with crystals just like you can communicate with the YOU-Niverse. After all, crystals are a part of the YOU-Niverse. You can communicate with a tree in much the same way. Ask a question with an empty mind, and then see or feel what the Universal Database brings to you. It may be a feeling, a knowing, or quite often you may hear a gentle voice, giving you an answer. All you have to do is trust, because sometimes the answer may not be logical or it may not be what you were expecting or want to hear.

I use crystals in my healing. Not always, but sometimes. I will create grids or geometric structures from them, in my healing space. When I do this it creates a vortex of energy in the room that I am in.

Here is a picture of one type of grid I use:

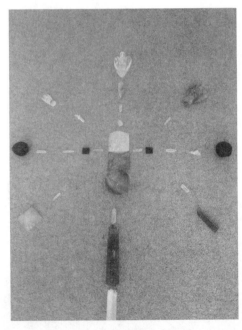

33. Geometric crystal grid

You don't need to use them but they can be fun to experiment with. It creates a different dynamic. I was shown how to create efficient crystal grids in the Ancient Mystery Schools of Egypt. There always must be a central point for the energy/light to flow to, and the crystal structure has to be designed in a way, that it brings in YOU-Niversal energy/light through an outer crystal layer, known as the generator.

It can take a little practise to harness the energy, and once you do, it will elevate the energy in your space tenfold. It's not a necessity to use crystal geometric grids; however, I strongly suggest you play around with them, and feel it for yourself.

When it comes to what crystals you should use, go with your instinct. I have a variety of crystals and go with my intuition every time. People will tell you that different crystals do different things but I simply listen to my heart and the rhythm of YOU-Niversal intelligence.

Once your Third Eye is functioning well, you will be able to see the light energy flow from the crystals in waveforms and see what each crystal's function is. You will then be able to communicate with the crystals to optimize their performance and effectiveness. This takes practise, an open mind and the willingness to let go and be childlike.

So how do I use these crystal grids?

I will have the crystal grid set up on the floor in front of me and I sit upright in my healing chair. I generally sit for distance healing. In a seminar or workshop I will always stand, but remotely I sit, 90% of the time, although I may stand during a session and then return to the sitting position.

So the human being I am facilitating the healing of will be in their space. I will bi-locate (being in one or more places at any one time) into their space. Once there I will then know what to do. Until a healing has started and I bring up the client's holographic blueprint I never know how the healing will pan out. It's always instinctive, based on what the hologram tells me. I may facilitate the healing there, or alternatively, come back into my own space, and work from where I am.

Both are just as effective depending on what is needed to be done. When you start playing a football match you can't tell how everyone will move, where the ball will be at every exact moment; you simply flow, react and move with the game. Star Magic Healing or Star Magic Information Exchange is the same.

When it comes to the crystal geometric pattern on the floor, this is what happens. I bi-locate into their space. Once there I pick their body up. Not with my arms but with my mind. I will levitate their body. It will rise up and I bring their body back into the space with me. Once back in my space their body will hover above the crystal geometric structure on the floor. The crystals on the floor will lock into the hologram, go to work and assist in the healing process.

I take my clients to other locations too. I will explain those later in the book. People often say to me that they felt their body floating, or their legs rose up in the air or, that they felt they were somewhere else. Some people describe the crystal structure, the surroundings, and some people will say I could see you looking down on me. Similar to when my friend saw me in her hospital room, in the UK, as clear as day, when really I was in New Zealand. Remember time and distance are illusions. The more you work with Star Magic, you will realize this by seeing and feeling it.

So as I am facilitating the healing and the crystals play their part, I can see what the crystals are doing. They work on the hologram the same way I do. There are streams of light emanating from the crystals and into the hologram, changing and manipulating the flow of energy and light, to create healing. I will be working on the hologram at the same time the crystals are.

Once you work with Star Magic long enough, you will be able to orchestrate an entire healing session without doing anything. *What do you mean, Jerry?* I can sit there and observe everything with my mind. I can move the light/energy with my mind and just sit there relaxed, as though I am the instrument being conducted in an orchestra. The light/energy is the musical symphony, I am the instrument and God is the composer. This takes practise and these techniques/ways are the most efficient and effective because you let go fully and get out of your own way, totally (advanced).

You will need to master the basics first. I want to highlight this point of basic, intermediate and advanced for you. Advanced is not more difficult to master than the basic technique or way. It's simply that by prompting the visualizations yourself (using basic ways) and you seeing and experiencing their effectiveness, you will then let go a little more and enable yourself to be a vessel or channel for consciousness to work through you.

You will integrate fully and become soul technology. You will allow higher-dimensional beings to play the piano or flute (you) and create a musical symphony from light codes, which in turn manifests in physical reality as what we may call energy healing. To be frank, I'm not sure if there is such a thing as energy healing.

Back to the geometric structure. So, I will keep the human being in the room with me until it feels I should take them back. It could be a minute or two or sometimes ten to fifteen minutes. I let the light dictate how the healing unfolds. It's the same as when a healing is about to finish. The client's body lets me know when it's had enough. My hands go even cooler and I just pop out (the best way to describe it) of my altered state of consciousness and I know it's time to stop. I seem to pop out of my trance state and be back in the room. If I have been paid for a certain amount of time I will often go over if the client needs a little more work. Again, I flow with the light. The energy/light is always sure. Not right but sure. Time and money can't end a healing session. Both are illusory, neither is intrinsic.

If you have never used crystals before, I suggest that you buy one or two. Go to a crystal shop and buy the ones you are drawn too. Hold them, feel them, listen to them and see what messages you can pick up. You can also buy clear quartz crystals on a pendulum for ten pounds or fifteen dollars. Hold it in your hand and shine light through it to cleanse it. You should always clean your crystals before using them, and periodically, once they are in your possession. Put them in the sunlight or moonlight, and now and again wash them in water. You can even shine light from your own body though your crystals to clean them.

Once you have bought your crystal pendulum, tell it that you would like it to answer some questions and that you would like it to spin right for yes, and left for no. You can hold the pendulum with the crystal dangling down. Make sure it's still. Then ask a question. Start with something simple. Is my hair brown? Ask some questions that you know the answer to already, so you can be sure the crystal is giving you the right information. Then you can start to ask questions that you don't know the answer too. The crystal will tell you. Your job is to trust.

Crystals are allies of the spirit world, intelligent and wise. Start getting to know a few and see where it leads you. The Egyptians used crystals a lot in their healing, and when we discuss the Pools of Consciousness later on, you will see how.

119

19

Geometry

When I engage with a client and drop down into the healing zone I will often experience geometric shapes such as the Flower of Life, Tree of Life, Merkabas (something that I utilize a lot in my healing) Metatron's Cube, Seed of Life, Pyramids and simpler shapes such as Triangles, Squares, Octagons. I also use the Full Christ Consciousness Grid in some healings. It's never planned but I go with the flow.

When I see these shapes I just know what to do with them. I will place them in certain parts of the client's body and watch them move, twist, turn and take on a life of their own. I never know what they are doing (logically) but they seem to create healing, and that is what matters.

As you are reading these pages, which have been infused with my consciousness, you will be downloading everything I know and see. So run with it when it happens in your healings. Don't think, *"Oh, what is that Triangle doing spinning on top of my right shoulder, that shouldn't be there."* Instead get curious. Ask yourself a great question such as, *"How can I use this triangle to instantly create healing in this human being?"* or *"Where shall I place this triangle or cube or Merkaba to create the most extraordinary miracle now?"*

Once you feel or see something, get curious and ask yourself empowering questions. Don't make dis-empowering remarks such as *"that shouldn't be there"*, because what will happen, if you do, is that you will create the reality without the triangle and then you will never know what magic the YOU-Niverse was trying to co-create with you.

Sometimes I will see a client's body in the formation of shapes. For example I had a client with a slipped disk. I didn't know it was slipped, she told me verbally she had a slipped disk. I had no proof it was slipped, I simply took her word for it. When I viewed her back I saw the issue as a series of Octagons where her spine was. Down near the bottom (I'm not going to give you a specific name for the disk, as I don't know) one of the Octagons was out of alignment with the rest. I decided to move it back in line with the others. When I spoke with the lady after the healing session she told me she was moving around like a twenty-year-old. She was in her sixties. Remember, imagination is reality.

20

Power Tools

I wanted to experiment with crystals and geometry one day so I bought a misty quartz pyramid. I contacted a friend of mine and asked him if he could help me create a healing tool or healing device. I was strongly guided to create this but needed an expert driller. My friend David was the man for the job. David creates powerful jewellery himself from various gems and geometry so I knew he would clearly understand what I was trying to achieve.

Once I had given David the pyramid we programmed it carefully with various metals and specific geometric shapes. This is what we used:

1 charged platinum capsule
2 times 9 carat gold triangles
3 silver spiral coils
2 disks with Metatron cube on one side and multi Metatron on the other
2 disks with the flower of life

We also used David's special technology to imprint natural botanic frequencies such as maca, aloe, vera and goji. This was processed into a special quartz powder and infused with the pyramid creating greater degrees of harmony with nature.

I remember getting the package through the post. I was just about to go out with my family. We got in the car and were driving down the road when I opened the package. The energy was phenomenal. I could feel it knock me for six. The kids and my wife started getting very nauseous. I had to put it back in the box and seal it up, as the energy was overwhelming.

The first night I kept it by my bed and couldn't sleep a wink. It was immense. I started using the crystal pyramid in healing sessions and it healed all sorts. I sometimes just get guided to use it. I don't know why, I just follow my intuition. It has a life of its own. A lady with arthritis came to see me. I got this little device out, aimed it at her knees and within fifteen minutes she was jumping out of the chair. I can see the waves of energy flowing from it, going to work but actually how this device heals I don't know.... Maybe the same way I do. Just by being there with my intention and pouring love onto the situation.

I wanted to see if I could make this device even more powerful so I input my own healing codes into it and programmed the crystal, with my intention, to use these codes as and when it sees fit. Remember the crystal is intelligent. It knows what to do. After programming the crystal with healing codes its ability to heal people was stronger.

I recommend you play and experiment with geometry and crystals. See what you can co-create. Follow your inner guidance. You will be amazed at what you can manifest.

21

Cellular Level –
A Little Deeper

When I am healing the holographic blueprints of others, to me, it is still fairly logical and it certainly has its place when it comes to Star Magic, and it will always have its place, because the visualizations do work, and work very well indeed. They are an integral part of the Star Magic remembering curve.

When you are working with Star Magic, the light/energy has the capacity to work on a cellular level. This enables me to release stuck emotions, blocks or traumas that the human being in question, could have been carrying for centuries, genetically, down through the lineage of their family. It's actually incredible that we, as a human race, now have the power, or should I say are aware of the power (because we have always had it – just forgotten it) to break the cycle. To break the emotional bonds that have caused mental and physical pain in this world, by using Star Magic. Star Magic is going to change your world, and everyone else's. Star Magic is going to change our world.

So when you are performing the visualization to facilitate the healing it still sometimes only removes the symptoms. It's one thousand percent better than any medical treatments, however, to be thorough, we must remember how to go deeper. The way I am about to share with you is one of my more advanced ways and this takes a lot of will power and mental strength. I do not advise using this method straight away. Get to grips with all of the visualizations; master those, play about with them, master seeing the specific holograms, geometry and explore your inner world, and then you can start going deeper. You will naturally go deeper.

This visualization involves taking people's bodies apart, to release the deepest fears and emotions. The ones that nobody wants to face. Firstly, this can be traumatic for the client. A healing process (some people call it a healing crisis but I don't like to use that term) happens afterwards, whereby these old blocks rise to the surface, to be observed, by the human being that is being healed. It can be a major roller coaster of emotions for days, weeks, and sometimes into months.

It's just a process, however, and it will pass. All things pass. There are people that by-pass all of this and the old stuff just shifts immediately. If this happens it is great. If you do facilitate the healing of someone that has to go through the healing process, if they request another healing to help them through this, in my experience, say no, and for very good reasons.

You can talk to them and support them but they must deal with this on their own. It's like a caterpillar inside a chrysalis. If you were to open the chrysalis too early, which scientists have done, the butterfly cannot fly. It is not strong enough. Being in the darkness, sitting and observing our emotions helps us grow. We become stronger. So allow your clients to go through this. Really and truthfully, it's a wonderful gift you are offering them. A blessing in disguise.

So, to get started, I will bring up the human being's hologram but in this instance, I will see this hologram as the client's real body. So in other words I am visualizing their body. I will always start at the feet. I place my hands on their soles.

To perform this you have to drop right down into the field, very deep indeed. When I put the intention to go deep, way down deep, into the cells to shift the genetic conditioning I see black energy fill the inside of the body. It's thicker in some places than others and I will do my best to explain this for you.

When you go this deep and are able to master this way, you will see that the majority of the body is black, that is because as humans, we have gone through thousands of years of stuff, mentally, physically, emotionally and spiritually and it's stored within our cells. Sometimes you will see some horrific sites, and the healing session requires pure mental toughness, to see it through to the end. Later I will share a story related to this in particular that details how difficult removing years of ancestral grief and human conditioning can be.

So place your hands on the soles of the feet, bring purple or violet light up through the Earth, through your feet and into your body. See it flow up through your legs and into your stomach. Bring white light down from the stars, through your crown chakra and let it meet the violet light from Mother Earth in the Centre of your body. See a vortex growing.

Now it's very important that when you do this type of healing, that your awareness keeps the two streams of light flowing. You cannot let the flow stop. You are going to need this powerful stream of light moving constantly.

On every healing you should be using YOU-Niversal light, and not your own energy, but this particular healing requires even more diligence. Remember, when using Star Magic we are working with light. We are not running energy as such, so you should never get depleted from this work. If you do then you need to check that you are working with streams of light that are coming in through the CNL.

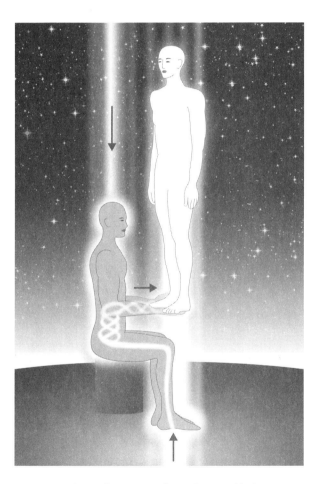

34. Channelling energy from above and below
through crown chakra and feet up through the healer's body
and into the human being

So the vortex is created and it grows within your body, and the light expands into all parts of your body, flowing down your arms and out through the palms of your hands, and into the soles of your client's feet. The light will also flow from your feet, into the human being's feet. And from your knees and other parts of your body. Once your Third Eye sight is functioning you will see this. Again I am offering you this way as a stepping stone to what waits for you later on.

22

Split Body Way

Now, continuing on…. what you will need to do is imagine the client's body being separated just above the knees. The knees carry so much emotion, and so do the feet and calves. What you are going to do is move the stagnant black energy from the soles of the feet, out through the top of the knees and into the ether, and see it being turned into pure white light.

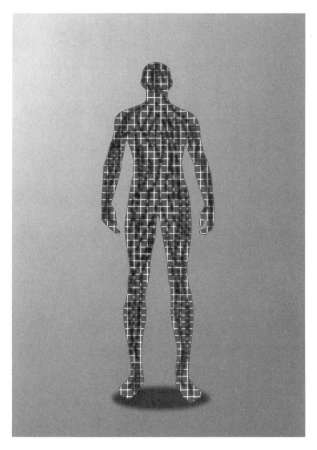

**35. Body with stagnant energy
(misty patches) all over**

If the top of the legs were there it can seem more difficult, only because of this 3D reality. Why make life difficult? Once you fully embrace the power of Star Magic, splitting the body will not be necessary but for now, trust me, take these steps.

Once you have cleared this area you are going to move the rest of the body back on top and join it back together again. As you do that you will need to seal the area you have just healed, so that old stagnant energy from the rest of the body, cannot flow back in. You do this with white light.

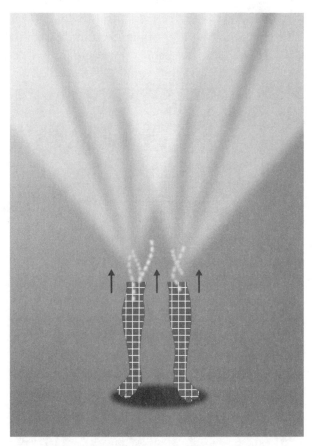

36. Healing the bottom part and releasing energy

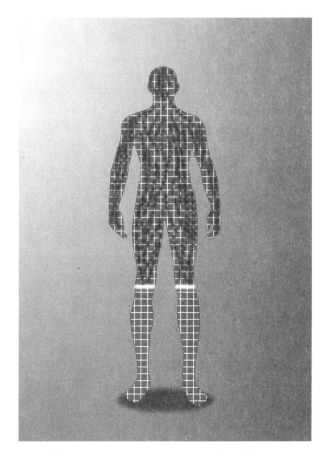

37. Legs cleared up to the knees; white light seal
to stop stagnant energy flowing back down

Once you have cleared up to and including the knees you then heal from the bottom of the thigh to just below the navel. You will repeat the same process. You remove the body from the navel upwards. Place it to the side, and allow the flow of light to work through your body and hands, up through the soles of the feet and into the legs. The journey of light through the bottom part of the leg will be easy, as you have already cleared it, and kept it clear.

You then see the light flowing up and pushing the stagnant energy from the legs, hips, buttocks and lower abdomen, out into the ether and turning into pure white light as it does so. The violet healing light then moves up to fill its place. You then move the rest of the body back on top and seal it as before.

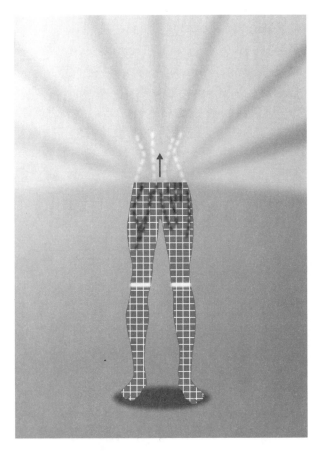

38. Lower torso with stagnant energy between
knees and navel before healing

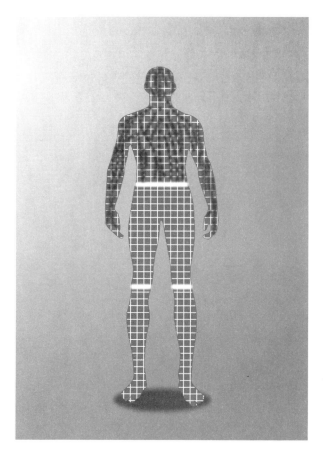

39. Body put back together with clear energy up to
the navel; seals of white light showing

Next you will need to remove the arms and the head and repeat the process. So this time you are healing/clearing the upper part of the body. The stagnant energy will flow out from the holes where the arms were and out from the neck. Remember you are still working from the feet. This is mission-critical as each time you are removing the next layer of stagnant energy, the entire body is being cleansed again and again. You then put the body back together again, sealing it so the upper body stays clear.

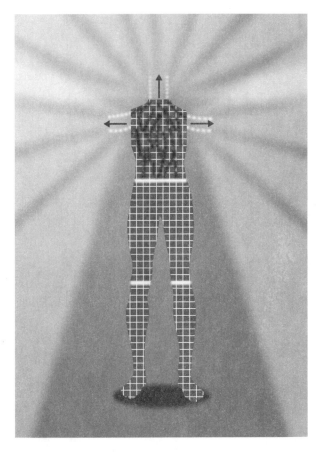

40. Arms and head removed, showing
stagnant energy releasing

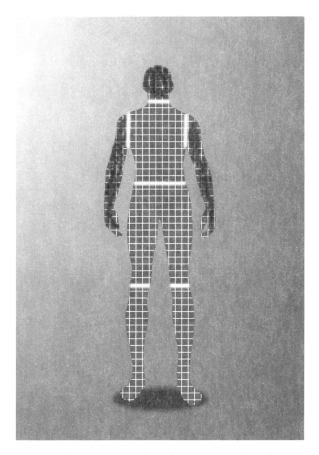

41. Body put back together, showing everything clear,
apart from the arms and the head

Next you will remove the hands and repeat the process. I always remove them at the wrists. Again, working from the feet, repeat the process. Once the arms are clear put the hands back on.

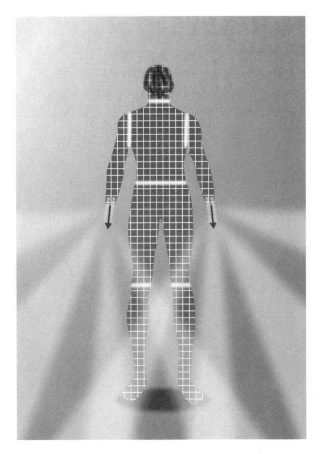

42. Hands removed, showing stagnant energy
releasing from the arms

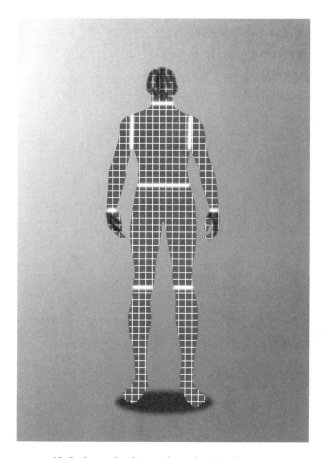

43. Body put back together, showing the arms
now clear

Next you will create a hole in the palms of the hands and the energy will naturally flood into the fingers and the rest of the hands pushing any remaining
stuck energy out from the hole in the palms. Keep the light-flow, through the
soles of the feet constant, until the hands are crystal clear. Again, ensure that
the stagnant energy leaving is turned into brilliant white light.

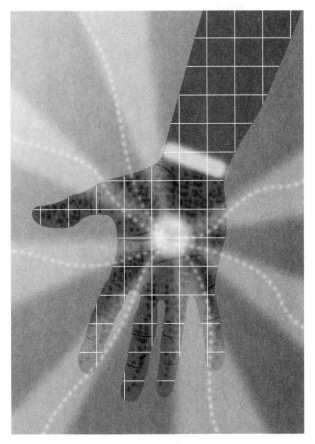

44. Energy flowing from the hand – hole in palm

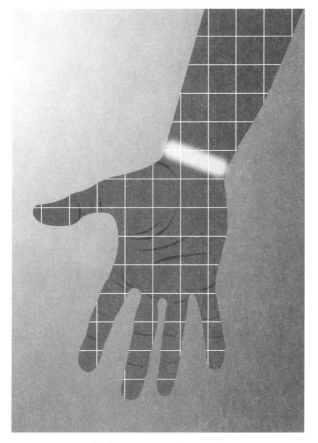

45. Clear energy afterwards

The final part is the head. This is always fun. The head is often clogged with so much stagnant energy. You will need to remove the top of the head and keep sending that light through the feet. As the light reaches the head, it will naturally spiral clockwise around the inside of the head. It is like it is scraping everything unnecessary from the inside of the head and sending it out of the top of the head. Once the head (and the entire body) is clear a beam of light will fire up and out of the top of the client's head with a mighty force.

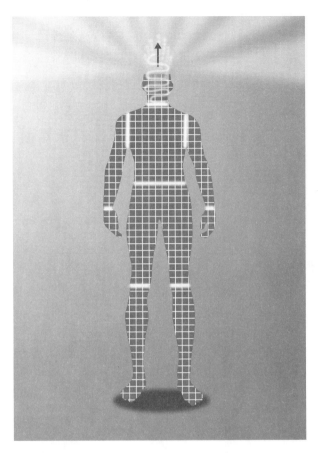

46. Top of head removed, with stagnant
energy flowing out

It's important that you keep the flow of light running strongly from the Earth, from the Stars and through your body, all the way through the human being that you are healing, and back out of the top of their head, and into the ether for at least three minutes.

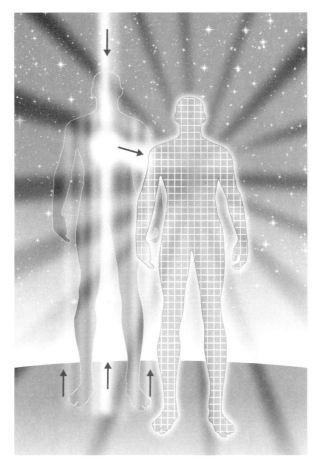

47. Light flowing from the stars and the earth through
the healer into the client and out into the ether

This entire process can take anywhere from five minutes to twenty-five minutes. It all depends on your mental strength and ability to move the stuck energy. I have seen some bodies with immense stuck or stagnant energy, and it takes a lot of effort, mentally. The resistance can be quite overwhelming at times and you must remain strong. When I perform this exercise in workshops people will often break down crying, as the emotional intensity of the energy (emotions) leaving, is overwhelming and powerful.

When this happens just accept it and go with it. Again, it's a part of the healing process. Sometimes the shift occurs and there is no emotional roller coaster. Quite often my clients will purge. If you have ever taken Ayahuasca then you will know what it feels like to purge on this level.

139

Below is the kind of message I receive after a distance healing session working on this level:

Dear Jerry,

Over the years I've had many a powerful healing session, which have left me feeling so washed out the next day, that I haven't been able to get out of bed – or alternatively I've had severe diarrhoea. But never have I experienced purging like this evening, as at 2120 hours. My nose and my eyes started running non-stop, and I began to feel nauseous, and knew it was time to dash to the toilet as I was about to vomit – which I did most prolifically – it just went on and on. I know this was a direct result of the Healing Session as now I'm absolutely fine.

I haven't vomited since 1984 and feel you have shifted some-thing at a very deep ancestral level, though emotionally it had no side effects on me – no flashback or painful memories surfacing, and it was very comforting knowing that I could contact you if necessary. Thank you for being there.

Love and Gratitude,
Chris xxx

I stress again that this way requires practise and you may not see the depths of the energy at first. You have to look past several superficial layers of toxicity, to be able to get to the core. You will do, you may just have to be a little patient with yourself. Drop down, trust, love and allow.

23

Clearing Pyramids

This way is again, advanced. The Egyptians used this a lot. They spent lots of time with me on this "way" in the Ancient Mystery Schools. I am not going to go into this way fully, as it would probably need an entire book of its own, which I will write, but for now I will give you something tangible that you can work with. When you are clearing old stagnant energy of this magnitude, you will, at times, face some serious resistance. I find it interesting, as I love a challenge, but you can, using clearing pyramids, make life easier for you. These pyramids will go to work for you. They work on their own, off the back of your intention, once you have set them in motion.

These pyramids are small. They are three-dimensional and out of each point you will see a stream of white/yellow light. This is what they look like:

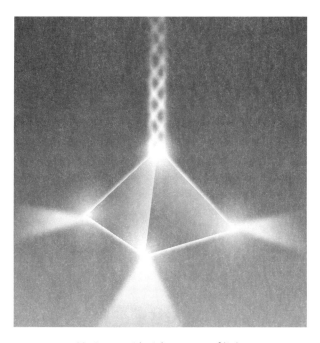

48. A pyramid with streams of light
whizzing out of each point

You will need to place your hands over the knees of your client, and you will see and feel the pyramids spring to life, or be born inside of you. They spring to life with your intention, inside your chest. They will flow down through your arms, out of the palms of your hands and into the person you are working with.

On entering their body the pyramids will go off and race around the body, breaking up any stagnant energy that needs clearing. They will race to every part of the body (with light spinning from each point) and when they have finished will return back through the knees, into your hands and back into your body. You must leave your hands, on or over the knees, whilst the clearing pyramids are working.

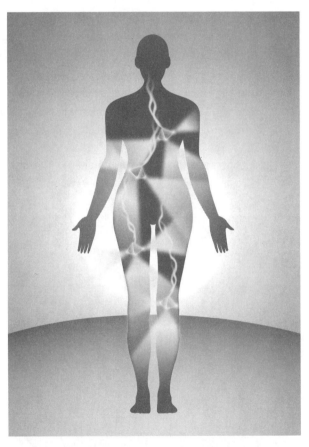

49. Pyramids racing around the body clearing
stuck energy with light streaming out

The clearing pyramids can only enter the body through the knees. Don't try other areas, it's dangerous. You have to be very careful with these pyramids. *They are powerful. Only use two.* Your clients will feel them racing around the body, and will see the streams of white light flashing through their mind. I will share with you how to use multiple pyramids for different circumstances in the next book along with a myriad of other uses for Clearing Pyramids. But for now practise with this. Trust me, you will get incredible results with this way.

One point I would like to mention. When the clearing pyramids decide to come back to your hands, allow them. They are like boomerangs. Leave your hands over the knees until they do return. Do not try and force them to do any more work. They know when they have cleared the space and shifted the energy, enough for you to go to work. Even if it looks like there is more they could do, do not force them. It's over to you now. They will have done enough for you to shift the rest.

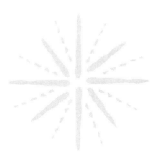

PART 4

24

Personal Team

This YOU-Niverse is multi-dimensional, and if you want to get to grips with Star Magic, and be the best Star Magic facilitator you can, you will need to realize that you are a small part of the Star Magic puzzle. The deeper you go and the further you travel on your Star Magic journey, the less you will do. I have a team that work with me. I have my personal team and I have my Star Magic Team (Star Team). You will have your personal team and you will also have access to the Star Team.

My personal team are a number of beings I have met on my travels. They are my multi-dimensional selves, and if you want to be the best you can be, it's important that you get to know these other versions of yourself, build a relationship with them and bring them home before each healing. By bringing them home, I mean bring them into the now, into your space, into your body, so you can align and be extraordinarily powerful.

You will meet these divine beings of light on your meditations or journeys, through the ether. If you want to know how I met mine I suggest you read my book *Into the Light*. Often they will come to you when you least expect it, or you can ask them to present themselves by using your intention. Meditation is another great way for communicating with them. You can sit in the quiet and ask out loud, or in your mind, *"Where are my spirit guides?"* or *"I would like to connect with my multi-dimensional selves, please come forth."*

I have a lot of Reiki instructors or healers using other modalities that come to me. They are amazed at my energy. They are blown away at the difference it makes to their healing sessions with their own clients. The reason Star Magic is so powerful is because I am using the full range of universal resources, and not limiting myself to my human body. Three perfectly aligned energy sources, are always going to be stronger and more durable than one, especially when we are talking on the level of these ultra-powerful, super-conscious beings of the spirit world.

We all were, at one point in space, completely whole and un-fragmented, and, as time has gone by, we have let other versions of ourselves go off on other journeys. It's time to bring them back and align with them. The following meditation will help in this:

> Close your eyes, take several, long deep breaths, and still your mind. Come into your heart and then in front of you see a door. Walk through this door and you will see a path on the other side. Walk down the path, through the grass, and you will come to a fork in the path. Take the path that goes to the right. Walk down until you come to a lake, a golden lake and around the outside of that lake you will see a large rock. Go and take a seat on it. Once you are sitting there, ask for your multi-dimensional selves to present themselves to you.
>
> They may come in the form of people or animals, angels or fairies. Have conversations with them, get to know them and let them know that you will be requiring their assistance in your healing sessions, and would they mind helping out. They are divine love and live in service. They will be glad to help you out. As soon as you request their presence, they are there. I see them all come into my space before a healing. They don't always all come, but the ones that are needed for the particular healing at hand, always come. As I am working on my clients they will be there too. People will often say, "Jerry, it felt as though there were several people in my room." And this is the reason why.
>
> Once you have spent some time by the lake you can make your way back the same way you came. Walk back though the door and into your space. This is a simple meditation to help you discover your personal team. It may take several journeys to meet them all. There isn't a specific number. You may not be ready to work with them all at once. Maybe you get introduced to one or two. When you are ready the rest will come. If you don't see anyone on your first meditation, that is OK. Accept this. Come back another time, and when the time is now, you will meet them.

Right time, space, sequence. Everything is always perfect as it is.

25

Star Team

There is a Star Magic Team. I call them the Star Team. They are the most incredible beings. I am going to introduce you to two of them. You will have to really let go of everything logical to work with these two members of the Star Team. I will tell you about them, and then share some words of my clients, who have been open enough to see them, during their healing sessions with me.

There is a Unicorn called Wisdom and a Pleiadian (the Pleiades are a cluster of Stars in the Constellation of Taurus and there is life there) called Rianar. These beings are multi-dimensional just like you and I, and have reached a stage on their spiritual path that is exponentially greater than ours – at present. Their capabilities are second to none. They are kind, honest, powerful and completely and utterly consumed by love. I met them during healing sessions with clients; they just appeared. It was at times when I wasn't getting the results that I wanted fast enough.

Then from nowhere they appeared and it just happened. When I say it just happened, I mean it was another kind of knowing. These beings appeared and then the healing took a different route. It felt right and I went with it. All of the time I knew I could stop what was happening, but I didn't. I knew it was divine intervention and this was something new/old I was remembering.

A client had suffered some extreme levels of abuse as a child and into her teenage years. It had caused a lot of trauma and suffering in her life. I was facilitating the healing and could see the stuck energy inside of her. It was so thick, like rock hard tar, or concrete. Not grey like concrete but as black as tar. I was moving this stuck energy on, clearing her out and it just kept coming back. As I cleared one layer, the next would appear and it just kept coming. I remember thinking to myself, *"I could do with a little assistance here."* And then I saw what looked like a lady with long blonde hair. I didn't pay too much attention at first, and then, as I continued the healing, she came right into my space. She then took my client's body onto an operating table in a space created from a light technology.

I will describe what happened next, the best I can. You know what an oxygen mask looks like? Well, it was as though she placed one of those over my client's mouth, but it wasn't an oxygen mask, it was more like a hoover or suction device. I was in a very futuristic environment, a spacecraft. She turned the machine on and it began to suck all of this black tar-like energy from my client's body. Huge amounts of it were being sucked out and into a holding tank – that is the best way I can describe it. I am not sure how long this went on for. I feel it was several minutes.

Once she had finished I could see the change in my client's hologram. The energy was completely balanced. The flow in the aura was perfect. There was no stagnant energy, on a cellular level, inside my client's body. It was incredible. Within a second we came back down into our space. She told me her name was Rianar, and will always be there if I need assistance.

After the healing session when I spoke with my client she said this:

> *Jerry, what happened? What did you see? That was very strange indeed. It felt as though something was inside of me sucking out my insides but I knew it was good. I knew it felt right. I could feel myself getting lighter.*

Before this healing Claire had been psychologically in despair. She couldn't cope with life. She had attempted suicide and was at rock bottom. After this healing, it was as though she had been given a clean slate. No more fear, no more trauma. No toxic emotions or ill feelings. She couldn't believe how great she felt and those feelings continued. They didn't subside in the slightest.

How is this possible? Because a being from another space came to help out with *Light* technology greater than our world knows. A natural technology, created by love. A super-advanced form of soul technology. I have learnt so much from Rianar. She has helped me in so many healing sessions. It's as though she is watching over me, and knows when I need her assistance. When you start to utilize Star Magic, the entire Universe will be at your beck and call.

I had another client who suffered from sexual abuse. I was facilitating a healing, and a unicorn came into our space. My client was on her bed. I was at home in my healing room but had bi-located to where she was, to facilitate the healing. I first took my client to Egypt (we will discuss this later) where my Egyptian brothers and sisters worked on her. We then came back into her space. These are Andia's words and a short account of the healing.

I was inside a chamber and these beings were all around me. They had created a structure of light around my body. It was like the most beautiful sacred geometry I had ever seen. They had rods of light, crystals. They were jabbing me. They were literally penetrating me with divinity.

This went on for several minutes. The next part of Andia's story that I will share is this. It's at this point that I met Wisdom, the second unicorn in the Star Magic Team. Alana was the first and we will discuss her another time.

I was lying on my bed. I have never seen so many beings present in my bedroom. This part of the healing was very traumatic but I knew it had to be this way. I was being thrown off my bed, caught in mid-air and then thrown back on the bed again. These beings were literally ripping black energy from my body. My room was filling up with it. I knew that this was the only way for these beings to get this out from my body.

It may sound a little far-fetched to some people. How could Andia be thrown off her bed, caught in mid-air and then thrown back on the bed again? When she was more than one hundred and twenty miles away, how? This is Star Magic. This is the power of the YOU-Niverse. We are not these little humans wandering around on a world, hovering in infinite space, all alone with no other life forms, and only this what is visible to most people's, three-dimensional reality.

Wisdom came to help with this healing and has been there for me ever since. She actually helps with every healing I do now. When you use Star Magic, you can call upon Rianar, and Wisdom for assistance. Just before you facilitate a healing, put the intention forward. Call upon these magical beings and let them know that if they feel they can assist you, then you will welcome their help. When you build your relationship with Rianar and Wisdom, the possibilities will open up and your healing potential will elevate.

Welcome to the world of Star Magic! As you go deeper and deeper and utilize Star Magic more and more I am sure the rest of the Star Team will introduce themselves to you. As you move across the levels, into new areas of potential (AP) deeper into unknown territory they will assist you when you least expect it.

26

Egyptian Pools
of Consciousness

I know that some of what I am sharing in this book will be too much for some people right now, and that using the basic ways will be as far as they go, and that is perfect if they/you feel this way. As you progress and start to integrate Star Magic into your self-healing, or healing facilitation practise, you will open up to the more mystical, yet very real aspects of Star Magic.

Some of you may turn around and say, *"But Jerry this is all a part of your imagination."* Yes, it is. But don't forget, your imagination is very real. And a question I would ask in return would be, *"What actually is your interpretation of imagination?"* Many inspirational human beings have shared the same views on imagination. Pablo Picasso said, *"Imagination is reality."* Albert Einstein said, *"Logic will take you from A to B and imagination will take you everywhere."* What is in your mind is a living reality. Your mind is taller than Everest and deeper than the Pacific Ocean. Start exploring.

If what I am about to share with you was just my imagination, how could other people experience it as I do? Surely, if imagination is something that just exists in our heads, or in this particular case, my head, how could others see the same? And not just see it, be in it? Since I visited the Ancient Mystery Schools my world opened up. I was taken to these healing chambers underneath the Pyramids.

I call them Pools of Consciousness because that is exactly what they are. There are several chambers way down deep, under the pyramids, and within them there are what look like swimming pools. They are not full of water however – but full of light/energy. In my group workshops I take people on guided meditations to bathe in them, and the experiences that take place are mind blowing.

There is a pool with a pure white light, and another pool with a violet light. There are others but these I use most of the time. During the facilitation of someone's healing I will bi-locate to their location, pick up their body, and take them into the Pools of Consciousness in Egypt. I will lay their bodies down in the chambers, and I leave them to float in the energy. Once they are there I can see the light go to work, and flow through their body. The actual part of the human being I take to the Pools of Consciousness is, I feel, the holographic blueprint. It doesn't actually look like the hologram does when I work at distance. It looks just like the physical body, but much lighter. Maybe, it's their soul?

Now what I don't understand logically is why the hologram actually presents itself to me as a life-like body, whenever I take my clients to the Pools of Consciousness. It always does though. What is even more interesting is that when I take my clients to this location, some of them can recall it. Accurately, down to the tiny details. Once we arrive in the chambers a team of very ancient beings come to help me heal. It's like I am a head surgeon leading a team to perform an operation.

These beings come out with crystal healing rods, and do what is necessary to perform the healing on my clients. They use a lot of geometry. They create geometric patterns with their crystal healing rods, and use them to send light through the human being in front of them. It happens very quickly.

Here are some comments from clients that I have taken to the Pools of Consciousness.

I floated out of my body. I was looking down at myself lying on the bed. Then I was covered in purple energy. It was beautiful. Then I drifted off and remember waking up in my bed.

— SARAH

I looked up and saw a team of what looked like surgeons. They were all around me working on me.

— MARK

I felt myself floating. It was like I was being dunked in the sea but it felt right. I could see purply violet colours surrounding me.

— JANE

There were these beings penetrating me with these rods. It felt very celestial. I could see them and feel them. I knew I was being healed at a deep level. It was amazing.

— CHRIS

I have had some very powerful healings over the years. I have travelled the world to see different healers. I'm seventy-two now and nothing has ever been this powerful. I don't know where you took me to Jerry, but the building was ancient and the energy there was truly amazing.

— ANDREA

Now when people have experiences like these, vivid recollections, you have to ask yourself, what is actually happening here? I have, many a time. I just come back to this phrase, *"rooted in love, not in logic"*. Logically it doesn't make sense. Well, actually let's look at this in a different way. Maybe logically it does make complete sense. Maybe it makes no sense in terms of what we have been taught is real or logical, and what is not. But in terms of the expansiveness and the infinite capacity of our heart and mind, and the capability they have, when combined, to access the spirit world, maybe, just maybe, Star Magic is opening us up to our true nature.

Maybe Star Magic is the key to Soul Technology. Maybe, all along we have been the technology but it's been kept a secret, because if everyone knew their own power, how would certain companies make their billions? Star Magic is giving you access to the other ninety-five percent of your human brain.

Something else that happens when I take my clients into the Pools of Consciousness is that Dolphins appear. Two of them. One will lie across the chest and one across the back with their bellies facing inwards. They shine love from their hearts; straight through the human being I am facilitating the healing of. When this happens in my group workshops, men and women will break down crying with tears of joy and happiness.

Often the emotions are uncontrollable because they have never experienced so much love before. Dolphin energy is so powerful. It's beyond description. When using Star Magic Codes of Consciousness (which I share later on), healing frequency (HF) 15 is Dolphin Energy. I can call upon the Dolphin Frequency at any time, not just in the Pools of Consciousness.

These Pools of Consciousness exist. There is many a secret I could reveal about what is actually underneath the pyramids. I've spent so much time exploring them. Remote viewing and bi-location is something that I have naturally been drawn to do. I am going to discuss remote viewing in the chapter called the "Secret Recipe", later in the book and explain how the military use it and how it explains a big part of what I do.

If you're a healer, you can take your clients to facilitate their healing there.

If your wish is to heal yourself, you can also take yourself there and facilitate your own healing. I explain that in the next chapter.

The infinite possibilities that lie within these Egyptian healing chambers are phenomenal. I have witnessed miracles happen. These miracles will now be a part of your life. I also feel that we are only scratching the surface right now with the potential of these healing pools. Everyday Star Magic is expanding within this field of unified light as my consciousness morphs and flows deeper into this electromagnetic wave of love.

27

Healing Visualization for Self-Empowerment

To be the very best facilitator you can be you must remove all blocks. The light/energy must be able to flow freely. So many healers work on others and neglect themselves. We all need healing, and, we are all healers. Work on yourself before you work on others. Or work on yourself in between working on clients. It is true that when you are facilitating the healing of another human being, you get healing too. With that being said, give yourself some undivided attention. You deserve it.

The following exercises will help you do this:

Mirror Image

Just like when you're facilitating the healing of someone else and you bring up their hologram, so can you do the same for yourself. Firstly, we all need healing, always. You can't have too much, so just like you brush your teeth each day, and take a shower, why not give yourself some healing.

You can imagine yourself in front of you. Just imagine yourself, as you are. The next thing to do is imagine white light coming down from the sky, and into the top of your head. See the white light travel down through your body cleaning it, and cleansing it as it goes, and seeing any darker energies moving out from your body as the clean energy passes through.

Personal Hologram

Try asking to see your own hologram. Just like when you are facilitating the healing of another, and you bring up their hologram, bring up your own. Trust that it is yours. You may question and say, *"Is this mine?"* Ask for yours and yours is what you will see. *"Please bring up the holographic blueprint of Jerry Sargeant."*

Then you can proceed to change the light in your own hologram, to remove energy blockages, and create an environment where self-healing can take place. You ask to be shown something you don't know that will enable you to facilitate the healing of this incredible human being. In this case, the incredible human being is you! Treat yourself just as you would another human being.

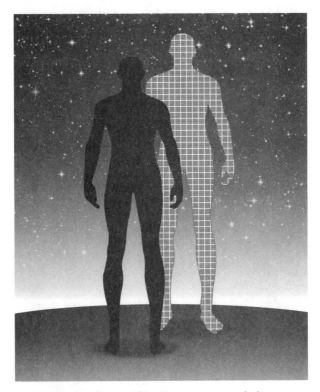

50. Picture of yourself looking at your own hologram

Star Light

Sit down or stand – it's up to you. If you can, do this standing, I find it much more effective. Imagine a stream of white light coming out from the top of your head and going up into the sky, way up into space. Once the stream of light is in space, see lots of smaller streams split off, and connect to different Stars in the sky. Ask to be connected to the stars, which will be best suited to heal and energize you in this moment. The streams of light will naturally go and connect with the stars.

You will then see and feel the energy pulsate down from the stars and penetrate your body. You will feel and see this Star Light energy, filling you up. Stay there for as long as feels right for you, and when you're ready, just undo the connection with your mind. This exercise is very powerful. You will also download information when you do this. Remember light is information.

Not from this world but information none the less. Feel it and slowly integrate it. A daily dose of Star Light should be recommended by every doctor to his or her patient.

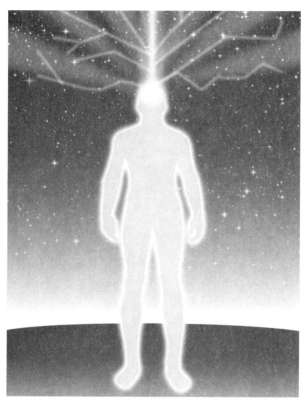

51. Star light feeding into the body

Pools of Consciousness – Self-Healing

I am going to tell you a story about a time that I healed myself in the Pools of Consciousness. One day, I was having a day where there seemed to be a lot of heavy energy around me. There are not so many light forces in this world and sometimes the darker ones will send low-vibrational frequencies to try and derail your train.

I call them shadow parasites. They are fourth-dimensional entities. They feed off of human fear, and try and induce it by sending low-frequency signals into your consciousness but you must know that love is the remedy. Remember that not all your thoughts are your own so question them. When you are journeying inwards on your spiritual quest, shadow parasites often try and affect you. They will, however, once you have ventured far enough into the light, leave you alone. It's like they have a healthy respect for you, and say, fair play – they've worked hard. They are in the light now – let's leave them alone.

So I was having one of those days. I knew what was going on and so I thought I will take a trip to Egypt. I envisioned myself in front of me, just as I would a client, and took myself off to Egypt. I put myself in the light, inside the Pools of Consciousness, within the healing chambers, under the pyramid.

I saw myself being healed. Beings were coming out and healing me and the light was pouring through my body. Now I am sharing this story with you because what happens next is truly fascinating. I am in my healing room, in my house, with my eyes closed and my wife calls me quietly, from outside the door. She knew I didn't have a healing session booked with a client at that time, but didn't want to disturb me too abruptly in case I was journeying, which I was. Nevertheless she wanted to talk to me.

Now, I could hear my wife calling my name, but I couldn't move. I was completely paralyzed from head to toe. I couldn't even open an eyelid. It was as though I was very far away. Which I was in my mind (and as it appeared my body too) – I was in Egypt. My wife left me alone, as she knew I was doing something and couldn't talk. So I brought my awareness back to Egypt. I finished the healing process and then brought my awareness back into my room. Once I was back I still couldn't move. I managed to open my eyes but was completely paralyzed (the only way I can describe it) everywhere else. I tried to shout to my wife or kids, whoever could hear, but my mouth would not move. The words were in my mind but I could not speak.

I just relaxed, accepted that I was going through this, and became aware of my entire body. I realized that I was still in Egypt being healed and because my concentration had been broken, when my wife called earlier, I came back too early. The healing was still being facilitated, even though I wasn't aware of it. And so I could not move my physical body. It was the most bizarre sensation. I didn't feel nervous and I didn't panic. I felt very calm but knew, I just had to sit tight. I am not sure how long it took for me to be able to move. It felt somewhere between ten and twenty minutes.

Gradually I could feel my body coming back to life. First I could move my head and, gradually, further down my body. My legs were the last to be able to move. It was strange. Once the rest of my body was freed from this paralyzed state, my legs were firmly stuck. Eventually they came around and I could move again. I just sat there in the chair. I felt on top of the world. I felt great. I was still trying to make sense of the experience.

Everything happens for a reason, and I feel that I was given this experience, so I could fully appreciate the magnitude of what takes place, in the Pools of Consciousness – and how real they are. The YOU-Niverse was allowing me to experience a full-blown Star Magic healing experience for myself.

This was the first time I took myself into these Pools of Consciousness and I have been back many times since. I have learned to trust the energy. Go with the energy. The light and the beings that are living in the space, of our beloved multi-verse, know what is best for you/us. You have to trust and go with it. Let go and feel. Let go and know. Let go and love. Clients often tell me that they are tranced out during a healing and come round but can't move. They describe it as being paralyzed too. I always run through this possible scenario now with everyone, just in case it happens to them as it seems to happen more and more often. It's actually a beautiful experience when you let go and accept.

I strongly recommend that you get to grips with the basics first. Start with simple ways, and once you have mastered them, you can try taking yourself to Egypt and bathe in the Pools of Consciousness.

Hemispheric Synchronization

We have a left and a right brain, male (left) and female (right). The male is logical and the female is intuitive. It's important that both hemispheres interact fluidly and are fully functional.

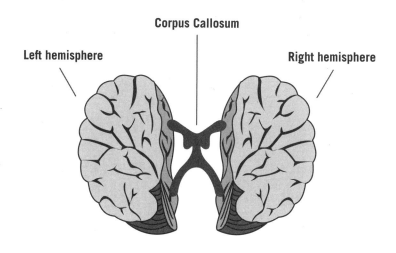

52. The two hemispheres of the brain with corpus callosum

When you work in both hemispheres your ability to connect, see, feel, know, heightens in the most extraordinary ways. By opening the channels of communication between these two parts of your brain and then combining this with pineal gland activation later on, your extra-sensory abilities will go into overdrive. Then all you have to do is trust.

The illustration on the previous page shows a bird's eye view of the two hemispheres: You will see the corpus callosum that links the two. This is the key. I want you to imagine white light coming down from the Universe, from outer space, from the stars and entering an upside down pyramid, which is hovering just above (9 inches) your head. See the light flow into the pyramid. The pyramid is spinning clockwise. It is bringing in more and more light and filling up. When you are ready, see that light flowing out through the apex of the upside down pyramid and piercing your corpus callosum.

It's best and most easily accomplished if you see the corpus callosum as a tube or tunnel. Once you see it as a tunnel you are entangling the two.

You may notice, if you haven't done a lot of work with light before, that the corpus callosum seems blocked. See the light filter into this area and break open any areas that are blocked. See the light move left and right, back and forth, clearing this passageway. The blockages disintegrate with the intensity of cosmic light. You then start to see the light flowing freely between the two hemispheres of the brain.

Once this happens and you practise regularly, you will start to see the world in terms of geometry. Boundaries will disappear. This will enable you to have more fun with Star Magic, as you will see the truth in all things. You will start to use more right brain to heal and the left brain to do some of the human things we do. Once the two are in balance, working in harmony, your life will never be the same again.

I actually visualize the link between the two hemispheres as a tube or a tunnel. It's easier to see the light pass back and forth. You are visualizing a tunnel and then entangling the tunnel and the real link between the two hemispheres with your intention.

Exercise to show the difference between two brain functions

Here is a quick exercise you can do to show the difference between the two brain functions. Bring your awareness fully into your left brain, the logical aspect. Then move it back to the right brain, through the corpus callosum. Do this three times. Spend 30 seconds in each side as you do. Once you have done this three times, move back to the left and stay there. Now, from your left brain take your awareness to your home. Stand outside your front door. Look at it. Then go inside and walk around. You will notice that it looks pretty normal.

Next, bring your awareness back to your left brain and then travel through your corpus callosum to your right brain, your female intuitive side. Now, take your awareness to your home. What can you see? Go inside and look around, spend a few minutes exploring. When you are ready bring your awareness back to your right brain, into the centre of your corpus callosum and then back into your body. You will notice that when you view your home from the right side of your brain it is hard to make out as everything is patterns, geometry, space. Here you see the truth. In my workshops I have a long version of this in a meditation. It's super-powerful. This is just a quick glimpse for you so you can see and feel the difference.

28

Healing Visualization
for Expansion and Growth

You are not your body. You are light and it's important that you enter a state where you are able to function as light, separate from your human body, as often as possible. The more often you drop into an altered state of consciousness, the faster your ability to facilitate your own healing, and the healing of others will occur.

Entering this altered state is something I refer to as "dropping in" or "dropping down". I am not sure why I call it dropping down. Maybe it is because I slow my breathing right down to enter this state. To bring my light, my spirit, out from my body, fully, I slow my heart rate down to around twenty-five beats per minute. I had an excellent role model on my spiritual journey, who taught me how to travel through other dimensions by bringing my light out from my body.

I remember the first time I did it. My heart rate slowed right down. I put my intention to move forward and I just popped out from my body. I turned around and looked at myself sat in the chair. To be in two places at once and be fully aware, was incredible. Strange, but incredible. This is a gift I utilize today on a regular basis.

So it's important that you remember, how to be just light, and leave the physical limitations of your own body behind. It's mission-critical that you can drop into the state of pure consciousness, source energy and move through space with ease and grace. For this, I am giving you a selection of basic visualizations/meditations/exercises that you can do to feel your light and move with it. See these basic exercises as stepping stones to fully bringing your light from your body. You may naturally go to the stage of fully separating from your body. If not, it's perfect. Be patient.

Energy Awareness

1. Breathe deeply for two to three minutes. Breathe in for five counts, hold for three counts and let out for five counts. Eventually you

will be breathing in for fifteen to twenty seconds, holding for fifteen to twenty seconds and letting out for fifteen to twenty seconds. Maybe longer.

2. Feel the energy inside of your hands. Bring your awareness there. Then do the same with your feet. Move around your entire body and feel the energy/light inside of you.

3. Focus on that energy/light, moving your awareness throughout your entire body, up and down.

4. Bring your awareness over your entire body and feel the energy/light inside of it. Feel your entire light energy body at once.

5. Feel it and go into the energy. Stay very relaxed as you do. Keep breathing deeply and slowly and breathe into every cell of your body.

6. Eventually you will start to vibrate as you do this.

Energy Expansion

1. Repeat steps 1 – 6 as above.

2. Stay in this aware vibrating state for several minutes. Feel yourself going deeper into your light/energy body as your physical body starts to feel numb.

3. Bring your awareness into the centre of your stomach. See a light, a bright ball of light that is brighter than the brightest star. Know that this light is a part of you.

4. See the light expanding. See it grow and start to move throughout your entire body, filling every cell as it moves.

5. Once your body is completely full from head to toe, with your mind, expand this energy. See and feel it move out past the boundaries of your physical body. See it expand and grow further in all directions.

6. Continue to see this energy grow larger than the room you are in. Taller, wider and more expansive than the building you are in or the outdoor location. See and feel this energy go out past your town or city and know that this is you.

7. You can play about with how far you expand your energy.

8. Stay in this space for however long you feel is right.

9. When you are ready, by engaging your intention, withdraw your energy. See and feel it becoming smaller until you are back to the small ball of light inside your stomach. Leave that ball there to glow.

Bird's-Eye View

1. Repeat steps 1 – 6 from "Energy Awareness".
2. Stay in this aware vibrating state for several minutes. Feel yourself going deeper into your light body as your physical body starts to feel numb.
3. Bring your awareness into your head. The centre of your head. Hold your awareness here for approximately one minute. You don't need to time it. Approximately. Until it feels as though you should move to the next stage.
4. Now bring your awareness to the top of your head, your crown chakra. Hold your awareness here for approximately one minute. You don't need to time it. Approximately. Until it feels as though you should move to the next stage.
5. Now bring your awareness about two metres above your body. You will be able to look down and see yourself lying, sitting or stood where you are. It's highly likely that you will still be in your body at this time but also hovering in the air (in two places at once but not disconnected). You will still be able to feel your body.

   When you completely remove your light from your body you can't feel it. If at this stage, you do pop out (the best way I can describe it) from your body, and there is total separation, just relax. It can seem a little strange the first time it happens. Know that you can go back by using your intention.
6. When you are ready, bring your awareness back into your body. Feel your hands. Feel your feet. Wiggle your fingers and toes and bring your attention/awareness back on to your physical body and feel it fully.

Practise with these basic ways as often as you can. The more you can feel this light and not feel your body, the deeper into the healing facilitation state (HFS) you are going. After enough practise you will be able to command this state in less than a heartbeat. It can take some time. Be patient if it does for you. On my workshops we live in this state and it is pure bliss. Hard to function 24/7 in the real world like it, but bliss none the less. It is the reason that so many people experience such profound shifts in my workshops. By being in this altered, deep state, miracles happen.

29

Meditation Techniques

If you want to harness the full power of meditation, you must learn to control your mind. Your mind is the second most powerful (your heart is number one) tool you possess. It can create harmony or total chaos – the choice is yours. If you let your mind run riot on its own your ego will keep you in the illusory world of the future and past and this, my friend, is chaos. By meditating, creating space, becoming still in your mind, you create a natural environment where your creativity can flourish and clarity takes over your soul.

Once you activate this sense of clarity and creativity, you will begin to see during your meditations and expansion exercises, that your ability to nurture the technology of your soul, Star Magic, happens much faster. Silence speaks. Silence contains wisdom. Silence breeds calmness and calmness is the trait of every great leader. A true leader can lead from a distance and as you develop your Star Magic ability, you will harness the Ultimate Star Magic capability.

That is to heal without doing anything. To facilitate the healing on a one-on-one, or a group level, from a place of complete stillness and expansive silence. By you harnessing your mind through meditation you will elevate your chances of mastering this skill. I am going to discuss this in detail later on.

So here are some basic meditation ways you can use:

1. Sit or lie comfortably. You may even want to invest in a meditation chair.
2. Close your eyes. Or have them open. There is no set-in-stone way to meditate.
3. Make no effort to control the breath; simply breathe naturally.
4. Focus your attention on the breath and on how the body moves with each inhalation and exhalation. Notice the movement of your body as you breathe. Observe your chest, shoulders, rib cage and belly. Make no effort to control your breath; simply focus your attention or just be aware. If your mind wanders, simply return your focus back to your breath. Maintain this meditation practise for 2–3 minutes to start, and then try it for longer periods.

Concentration Meditation

A concentrative meditation way involves focusing on a single point. This could entail watching the breath, repeating a single word or mantra, staring at a candle flame, listening to a repetitive gong or counting beads on a rosary. Concentration meditation is an excellent stepping stone to set you on your path.

In this form of meditation, you simply refocus your awareness on the chosen object of attention each time you notice your mind wandering. Rather than pursuing random thoughts, you simply let them go. Through this process, your ability to concentrate improves and eventually you go past concentration and into full-blown awareness. Don't stay in concentration. It's important that you know awareness is the way. Concentration is a stepping stone. Awareness sits just behind concentration. It's the underlying essence of concentration. It's the underlying essence of all things.

Mindfulness Meditation

The word mindfulness is thrown around a lot these days. It implies the mind is full. What we want is an empty mind. To create an empty mind, again, mindfulness is a stepping stone. This meditation way encourages the human being to observe wandering thoughts as they drift through the mind. The intention is not to get involved with the thoughts or to judge them, but simply to be aware of each mental note as it arises.

Through mindfulness meditation, you can see how your thoughts and feelings tend to move in particular patterns. Over time, you can become more aware of the human tendency to quickly judge experience as "good" or "bad" ("pleasant" or "unpleasant"). With practise, an inner balance develops and labels disappear. In life and Star Magic, as well as meditation, observation is the key.

Light Meditation

A great way to meditate, and this helped me so much, as I was trying to still the mental chatter. Every day I went into meditation I focussed on a light at the front of my head. Just between my eyebrows and up a little. In the area of your Third Eye. Close your eyes, focus on the light and breathe. Allow the light to take you on your journey – wherever that may be.

Meditation to Breathe

Focusing on your breathing is simple and so effective. Follow your own breath, in and out of your body. Every time your mind wanders, bring your focus back to your breath. Breathe deeply into the pit of your stomach and let the breath out slowly.

Tree Meditation

Why not go into nature, sit by a tree, or even better, cuddle a tree and feel its light/energy. Breathe slowly and open your heart. Feel and see light coming from your heart and into the tree whilst you breathe and cuddle it. By opening your heart and having your awareness on your heart chakra, your mind will be still. If it starts to chatter, say thank you and come back to your heart.

There is no right or wrong way to meditate. Find what works best for you. I like to be in nature, by water, but I also like to meditate in very busy places. We must be able to meditate in the middle of Times Square or Piccadilly Circus. If you hear noise when you meditate, whether it's a car or a bird, or a human talking, go into the sound. Use the sound to go deeper. Everything can be used to your advantage.

Sometimes, when there is a stream of incessant thoughts, in or outside of meditation, you can create space in your thought stream, very quickly, by asking yourself a very simple question. Here it is:

"What is the next thought that is going to come into my head?"

Once you have asked yourself that question watch your own mind. You will see that instantly your thoughts stop and complete presence occurs. You enter the now as an observer. This is meditation. No images. No thoughts. No ideas. You can access this at any time. Try it now. Ask yourself, *"What is the next thought that is going to come into my head?"* Interesting isn't it how the mind stops. It won't stop forever but it gives you space. The more often you invite space into your life, the quicker you connect with the essence, that allows Star Magic to flow through your consciousness, allowing the clarity, connection and free flowing healing juice to run through your veins.

Heart Connection Meditation

I love this meditation. I run a Global Meditation Group every Wednesday and often we stop, as a group, join our energy fields together through our heart and shine love over this beautiful planet. It's so powerful. I will give you a very short version of this meditation that you can do on your own.

Breathe deeply and come out of your head and down into your body, bringing your awareness into your heart space. See a beautiful crystal white coloured light filling up the inside of your sternum. Keep breathing as it fills up, getting brighter and stronger. Once the inside of your sternum is filled with this bright light, with your intention, open your heart and see this beautiful light flood outwards and into the YOU-Niverse.

See it flow out of the back and the front of your heart chakra. See and feel this light flow further than your imagination, in all directions, connecting you to everything. People, animals, flowers, plants, trees, insects, rocks, the sun, the moon, the stars, planets – a bright crystal white blanket of love-filled light, coats the entire planet, connecting you with everything, through the vibration of love.

Spend a few minutes, or as long as you feel is right for you, feeling unified, at one with all life everywhere, all creatures great and small – all sentient beings. Connect to every human being with that feeling of unconditional love. Being on this vibration will create the perfect environment for Star Magic to flow. After all, Star Magic is rooted in love, not in logic. Healing takes place in your heart, not in your head. Miracles are born of the heart and obstructed by the head.

Stay in this space, feeling connected, pouring your heart out to the planet and beyond. Feel and be this connection. Remember, the love that pours from your heart is in infinite supply. It can never run out.

> *I invite you to join our Global Meditation Group. Please visit* **www.starmagichealing.com** *and register. Each week I will take you through a powerful guided meditation, in our virtual meditation room. The meditation is infused with Star Magic healing frequencies. People call in from all over the planet. It's beautiful.*

30

Guided Meditation to the Crystal Temple of Joy (Atlantis) – 12D Light

Start by sitting, lying or standing. Your eyes can be open or closed. Take several long, deep breaths and let them out slowly.

See a golden bubble come into your space and surround your body. Coming into this bubble are the energies of Atlantis. The colour is electric blue. Breathe this electric blue energy into your body. Into every cell, until your body is full.

Bring in this intention by using the following mantra:

> I [name] choose to accept and integrate, a deep illumination of the 12th Dimension of Christ Consciousness. I also bring in the Gold Ray of Christ, and the Atlantean Ascension Energy, within my Merkaba and complete Christ Consciousness Grid Structure... thereby allowing a full, open manifestation of my Divine Ascended Self in service to Gaia, humanity and All That Is.

Feel this energy flowing through your being and be aware of the Star Energies of the upper dimensions filtering through your consciousness.

Illuminated Dragons are now joining your space to guide you on this journey. Allow them to guide you and share their healing energies with you. See and feel them breathe their flames of protection all around you.

Then become aware of a door. Walk through that door. On the other side you will be in a field, with a path. Start to make your way down the path. Feel the love in this environment. See and feel the vibrations in all that is, the flowers, the insects, the trees and the animals.

In the distance you will see the Crystal Temple of Joy. It is way up high upon the blue mountains on the Island of Poseida. Poseida was the home to many great priests and priestesses during the Atlantean Era. You will feel the energy here is not like on Earth. From here on in you will be receiving a powerful download and frequency upgrade. Welcome it.

As your Dragons guide you down the path, light/energy is flowing into your being from everything within this environment. You are fully aware of one unified field of cosmic light, which you are a part of. Zero separation.

As you approach the bottom of the mountain two Unicorns are waiting for you. They bow their heads, place their horns inside your heart chakra and penetrate you with divinity from their horns. Your body starts vibrating as this energy flows through you, running deep into the core of your being. No one has to say anything. You are downloading with an internal knowing.

The path that leads up the side of the mountain is made of a pure brilliant white marble. You make your way up it, accompanied by your two Unicorns and the swirling Dragons. The mountain is four hundred and forty-four metres in the air.

Once you reach the top you are in awe of this beautiful sight in front of your very eyes. You are told by your Unicorns, guardians of this temple, that today you will be introduced to the full-blown power of your own Internal Light.

On the door to the Temple is a number Nine. You walk up to the door and are greeted by Giantriva, a Goddess of Atlantis and keeper of the temple of joy. She has golden light emanating from her, pouring out from around her. She welcomes you inside.

Once you enter the temple, which is in the shape of a pyramid, a clear quartz pyramid, you find a place to sit down. There are crystal thrones everywhere. You find the one that feels right for you. You place your arms in the rest and at the end of each of the armrests are two crystal handles. You place your hands around them, and the light starts to flow through your hands, up through your arms and throughout your entire being. You become crystalline. Totally pure. All you can feel is unconditional love, for all beings in the Universe, and a deep love for yourself

Inside the temple it seems to be like a community of divine light energy forms; floating, moving effortlessly, watering flowers, communicating telepathically, in harmony with one another. No verbal communication and everyone seems to just know. A flawless community, living in harmony with one another and their environment.

The walls of the temple are clear. You look out at the breathtaking views all around you. It's stunning.

As you continue to sit down in the chair, now a part of the chair and the temple itself, you start to download wave after wave of light. Light is information; information from the upper dimensions, nine, ten, eleven and twelve. You can control this download. If it's too much, ask to slow it down. If you want to speed it up then do so with your intention.

Once you have downloaded as much light energy as you require, a beautiful angelic lady, comes towards you. She leads you up a golden staircase. When you reach the top there is a crystal bed, within the apex of the pyramid. You lie down and relax, looking out for miles around. You can see the oceans, the beaches, the lush forests and the clear blue skies. Giantriva is sat in a chair, overseeing everything that is happening. You relax and rest.

The bed is directly underneath the apex of the pyramid. It is drawing in light and sound codes. It's drawing in Star Magic from other worlds, the stars and multiple Universes beyond ours. This light and sound flows through the apex of the pyramid and penetrates your Third Eye, like a laser beam of divinity.

These codes trickle and flow through your cells, upgrading your DNA. You now tune into:

- The Light of The Pleiades
- The Luminosity of Orion
- The Deep Knowledge of Sirius
- The Ascended Aspects of your own planetary systems
- The 9D light of the Galactic Spiritual Suns…Helios and Vesta
- And most prominently, the 12D light of Bevricon.

There may be, and probably will be, others that come to you also… be open and ready to receive this divine extra-terrestrial light. Let go and feel. Don't try and understand, simply allow.

Feel all of these light codes integrating, and activating the blueprint for your Higher-dimensional Cosmic Master Self. You, after all, are an ascended master. You are coming back home.

As you relax and let go you will get brighter, stronger and feel your true power, your divinity and wholeness. Connections to all corners of the Multiverse have always been within you. Feel this deepest integration. Allow your light to expand, and transcend all boundaries of conscious reality. This field of light penetrates the core of your being. With every vibration, you remember more. Truth and divinity. At this moment, right now, you are All That Is. You are the almighty I AM presence.

Hear Giantriva in the background – talking or transmitting words of comfort and wisdom. She is acknowledging your divinity. You are now the Master of Light that you always were. There is no turning back. All of your multi-dimensional selves have returned to you.

You then begin to float, out through the apex of the pyramid. You float into the air and are met by your Unicorns and Dragons. You float back to the bottom of the mountain, effortlessly as pure consciousness. Once on the ground your heart chakra opens up. Both Unicorns place their horns inside and you can feel an electrical charge of love pour into you. It's their gift to you for coming on this beautiful journey and downloading this information, to share with the rest of your brothers and sisters, on our beautiful big blue Planet Earth.

You say thank you and goodbye, knowing you can return at any time you wish. One of your Dragons leads you back down the path to the door. You move inside and back into your space to integrate with your human body once more, bringing all of this divine wisdom with you.

Feel your body fully. Take your time. Count from five back to zero and when you are ready, open your eyes and come back into the space.

INSTRUCTIONS: Do this meditation as often as you wish. Each time you will download more information. The YOU-Niverse will give it to you as and when you are ready. Be open to receive and control the download at a rate in which you feel comfortable.

31

Pineal Gland Activation

Wikipedia defines the biological aspect of the pineal gland as "a small endocrine gland in the vertebrate brain. It produces the serotonin derivative melatonin, a hormone that affects the modulation of wake/sleep patterns and seasonal functions. Its shape resembles a tiny pine cone (hence its name), and it is located near the centre of the brain, between the two hemispheres, tucked in a groove where the two rounded thalamic bodies join."

Wikipedia also notes that it is also called the pineal body, epiphysis cerebri, epiphysis, conarium or the Third Eye, with the latter being the aspect most spiritually minded people focus on. This Third Eye activates when exposed to light, and has a number of biological functions in controlling the biorhythms of the body. It works in harmony with the hypothalamus gland, which directs the body's thirst, hunger, sexual desire and the biological clock that determines our aging process. All in all, a very important gland!

For a long time, the biological role of the pineal gland remained unknown, but mystical traditions and esoteric schools long held this area in the middle of the brain to be the connecting link between the physical and spiritual worlds. In the spiritual aspect, it is a necessary step to awakening the Third Eye, which will feel like a pressure at the base of the brain. It is important because activating it raises one's frequency and moves into higher consciousness – all is a consciousness experience perceived through the Eye of Time or Third Eye.

The Third Eye is considered the most powerful and highest source of ethereal energy available to humans, and because of this, the pineal gland has been seen as a gateway that leads within to inner realms and spaces of higher consciousness. Awakening the Third Eye acts as a "star gate." So how do you activate it? Meditation, visualization yoga, and all forms of out of body travel open the Third Eye and allow a human being to see things that are beyond the physical.

The key is Star Magic. You must invite Star Light, encoded with Space Geometry, through the ether and into you. You can bring this light in through your head or through your heart. It's irrelevant. Once it arrives, containing the formula of ascension, the power to unleash your full human potential, by upgrading the level of information flowing through your CNL, it will elevate your life by changing the infinite degrees of your human perception.

A list of the benefits and abilities the Third Eye brings include clarity, heightened awareness, perspicuity, bliss, intuition, decisiveness and insight, as well as:

- Vivid/Lucid Dreaming.
- More effective astral projection.
- Better sleep quality.
- Enhanced imagination/ability to see the truth.
- Enabling Aura viewing, seeing energy, seeing beings, and seeing with eyes closed.
- Clear channels and ability to feel light/energy more efficiently.

All of the above are key components of Star Magic.

However, if a human being is not taking care of their Third Eye, all of this is cut off from them. Calcification of the pineal gland will definitely occur without regular detox. Most people's pineal glands are heavily calcified by the time they are seventeen years old, so much so that they show up as a lump of calcium during an MRI. Calcification is the build-up of calcium phosphate crystals in various parts of the body. A closed Third Eye is no joke. In Hindu tradition, it is known as "Anja Chakra" and is credited with bringing confusion, uncertainty, cynicism, pessimism, jealousy, envy and one sidedness to a person's life.

The good news is that there's something you can do about it. Just because your pineal gland is calcified doesn't mean the door can't be reopened. With continual care and discipline, you will free your pineal gland in no time.

Your Third Eye is known as the seat of the soul. It gives you, when open and functioning, a view of reality that is real. Your two eyes that are located within your eye sockets filter information, then through your brain, it is filtered even more. We see a very small slither of what reality truly is. In fact, our human body is how we interface with each other or better described, how consciousness interfaces with consciousness. What we actually see through our eyes is not reality at all. It's what we have been conditioned to see reality as.

I have done a lot of work when it comes to operating with my Third Eye. It allows me to see the world in terms of geometry, patterns, light and sound and to understand the information that is contained in all that I see and feel. To properly harness the full power of Star Magic you will need to do the same. Star Magic will still work without your Third Eye sight but why would you want to miss out on seeing the truth and beauty that lies beyond the illusion?

Through life, growing up, your pineal gland has been calcified, just like mine was, and most other people's is. Through television, sugary foods, cans of pop, hormones and additives found in processed foods and what I call empty foods (genetically modified foods that look like foods but are not – which are sold in most large, mainstream supermarkets), toothpaste, tap water and some bottled water, contains ingredients that calcify your pineal gland, such as fluoride (found in public water systems and toothpaste). There is some speculation that cell phones are also part of the problem, thanks to high concentrations of radiation.

You have to ask yourself why would food be created that stops you seeing the truth? Well maybe, just maybe, it benefits a few shady characters if they can keep you dumbed down, on a low vibration, glued to the false reality, portrayed through the TV, the doom and gloom in the national press. Or the false hope of one day becoming like your favourite celebrity or X-Factor champ, or when your Euro Millions ticket drops a winner, as you continue to drink beer and pour M & M's down your throat, being excited about your Saturday night pizza or Chinese take away, and your Sunday morning happy drive-thru meal with the kids.

Life, when seen through your normal pair of spectacles is extremely limited. When you view life through your Third Eye, you see no boundaries. When I look at the YOU-Niverse through my Third Eye, I see one complete energy field. There are no humans, no trees, no buildings, no cars, no birds. I see a constant stream of light. It's seeing the world this way that opens up the full range of Star Magic abilities.

To fully appreciate Star Magic you must start today. You must start to decalcify your pineal gland and open up your Third Eye fully. At first it may not be nice. You may freak out. You will realize that everything you have ever been taught or made to believe is real, is complete B......S.

Now, when you do realize this, there is no one to blame. You must take full responsibility for buying into this façade. Your parents bought into it and so did their parents and so on. It's been going on for thousands of years. Change is always a little messy to begin with – just run with it. Sit in the mess until the fog passes, the mist rises and the sun slowly pours out over the mountaintop of love. So how do you decalcify your pineal gland and start to activate your Third Eye?

1. Eat natural foods – raw is best. Plenty of greens. Kale, spinach, avocado, green beans, broccoli. Berries are great, loads of berries. Raw Cacao, Goji berries, raw honey (not the stuff in jars or bottles), juice in the morning (fruits 20% and vegetables 80%), garlic, hemp seed, coconut oil, seaweed.
2. No more tap water. Filter your water and then charge it with love. You can find a template for a water charging symbol on page 247 of this book. Please cut it out, photocopy it and stick it to the side of a load of bottles. Fill these bottles up with filtered water and then leave them for two days before drinking it.

    This symbol will change the molecular structure of your water and charge it with love. It will fill the water full of love and dissolve the fluoride and other chemicals in it. Even showering without a filter has a detrimental effect.
3. Don't use regular toothpaste. It contains Fluoride. Find a toothpaste that doesn't contain Fluoride from a natural food store such as The Wholefoods Market.
4. No packaged foods.
5. No sugar or sugary foods.
6. No fast foods.
7. Meditate Daily.
8. Yoga.
9. Deep breathing always.
10. No TV.
11. No screens at all within an hour of going to bed.
12. No newspapers.
13. No radio.
14. Be off your phone and away from it as often as possible. Put it in airplane mode when you sleep and turn it off. Do not carry your mobile right on your body if possible.
15. Less time on the laptop.
16. Cuddle some trees a few times every week. Be in nature.
17. No alcohol or cut it right back.
18. Exercise. Walking. Jogging. Join a gym. Swimming. You're spoilt for choice.

It will, I know, take TIME adjusting for some of you. It took me a while to make these lifestyle changes. You have to ask yourself though. Do I want to live my one shot at this life, seeing only a small slither of what is available to me? Or do I want to fully experience this beautiful opportunity to live my life as a human? You're a spiritual being having a human experience, why not have that experience, fully?

19. Go into a dark room and close your eyes. Gently massage the spot between your eyebrows and up slightly. By stimulating this area, you will start to feel the tingles and vibrations of energy there. You can then focus on your breathing and be aware of what you are feeling.

   What do you see? Where do you travel in your mind? At first you may not go anywhere and that is OK. Be patient. Next, you will start to drift through other dimensions or maybe other spaces within this dimension.

   Eventually you will be able to direct your consciousness and travel wherever you want to go. I have practised this for years. I can go anywhere now. Government buildings, other planets, any location I choose. The more you explore the greater your ability will become.

   You can connect with beings in other worlds. Extra-terrestrials, angels, fairies, unicorns. They are not fantasies. They are real. As real as the pages you are staring at right now, or the Kindle or I-pad screen.

   I have been taken up in a spaceship before, as you know. Earth is a grain of sand compared to the magical, mystical, multitude of galaxies and YOU-Niverses out there. And are they really out there?

   Maybe they are in here? It could be that you are the YOU-Niverse and so contain every planet, universe and galaxy within your own DNA structure. Wouldn't that be something?

20. Another great way to activate your Third Eye is to sun-gaze. The first and last rays – when the sun is not too strong. Go and open your eyes and stare at it. Just for five seconds in the morning and evening. The next day do ten seconds and build up. The light will nourish you.

There are other more advanced sun-gazing techniques but this is enough to get you started. Ensure you are barefooted with your feet on the Earth if possible.

21. Chanting is a great way to activate your Third Eye. When you are sat in the dark, bring your awareness onto the area of your Third Eye and then chant the sound OM. But say it as AUM. You can also chant Allah. Say it as AAA –LA.

Also, this famous chant is incredible:

HARE KRSNA HARE KRSNA, KRSNA KRSNA,
HARE HARE
HARE RAMA, HARE RAMA, RAMA RAMA,
HARE RAMA

When you chant these keep going and focus on your Third Eye. It will start to vibrate like crazy. Try all three. They may all work for you or you may have a favourite. I have worked myself into a vibrating frenzy at times with these and popped straight out of my body. It's truly beautiful.

These are some tips to activate your Third Eye. If you want to be a Star Magic Facilitator this isn't a necessity but it's great to see the world beyond form as it makes healing more interesting. If you struggle developing your Third Eye sight it will not make your healing abilities any less potent. I want you to know however that you can activate your Third Eye sight. Everyone can.

You cannot shirk your responsibility when it comes to homework. This part of your study, this element of remembering, is very important. It is probably more important than any other part. Without your Third Eye sight you will miss out on the beauty of the world of formless form. Discipline is the key.

As the old saying goes, practise makes perfect. Well, you are actually perfect already so refine your levels of awareness. Practise is mission-critical however.

32

Quantum Knowledge

Everything in the YOU-Niverse happens now or is happening now. This means that you have access to everything there ever has been, everything there is, and everything there ever will be… now. Not tomorrow, next week or next year, but now.

If you want to access the skill-set of another healer, a sportsman, a speaker, actor, photographer or anyone else you wish; you can do so by entering the field now and downloading the light codes that contain that human being's personal experiences or specific skill sets. It's a bit like Neo in the film, The Matrix, when he downloaded his fighting skills. You just put the intention forward and plug in.

It's a bit like when I switched my client's legs for Usain Bolt's legs. They were healed. Once, I was viewing someone's Hologram and I could see that the spine was disjointed. I wasn't being shown how to correct it though. There was no movement in the Quantum Realm and everything seemed stagnant. I asked to be shown what other resources I had at my disposal and then St. Germain popped into my consciousness.

He is an ascended master, a little like Jesus, from what I understand. So I asked, *"What would you do in this situation, mate?"* as though he was my good old friend I hadn't seen for a while. *"Stretch her left leg"* was the reply. So I leaned forward and in my version of reality held her foot tightly and tugged on it. I pulled and her leg seemed to get longer. As it did, her hip seemed to drop down and her spine re-aligned.

I instantly popped out of my healing zone and into a full conscious state. When I spoke with the lady afterwards she could stand upright and there were no issues. Six months on she is still feeling like a new woman. I used the resources that are available to me as a human being and they are the same resources that are available to you and everyone else on this planet.

One day a young man got in touch who had been attacked in a park and had terrible recurring nightmares. He kept replaying the event over and over in his dreams. I first used a time travel "way", which we will discuss in the next chapter – which the majority of the time works – but in this particular instance it didn't.

So I asked my guides… *"What can you show me that I don't know, to ensure this man sleeps well at night?"* A picture of Bruce Lee beating up ten or so guys in Enter the Dragon popped into my consciousness. So I went back to the time travel way. I went back to before the man was attacked and down-loaded light containing the codes of Bruce Lee's skill set into his biological computer, his brain. Then the healing seemed to finish: quite abruptly. I was back in the room, out of my altered state of consciousness.

I spoke to the man again two days later. He said that he was still having dreams but this time he was winning. He walked through the park, was attacked and managed to floor all of his attackers. What is even more inter-esting is that within a week, every time he had the dream, he would walk through the park and no one would bother him. Now, he doesn't have the dream anymore.

I don't know how this works but it does. Does it matter that I don't know? No! Because it works. It may actually work because I don't know. Explore the infinite sea of possibilities and you will find the answers; always! You can jump through the Quantum realm and meet anyone you like, dead or alive. The ones that are dead are not really dead, not in the Quantum realm anyway. Everything is now and is readily available.

I often have "boardroom business meetings" with human beings that can help me or give me great advice. In my boardroom meetings I will invite Bill Gates, Will Smith, Albert Einstein and whoever else feels right at the time. The conversations are incredible. Explore your imagination and move through the space between space, meeting, greeting, inquiring and playing and you will open up the door that contains beauty, wonder, excitement, fun and the answers to all of your questions. Here you will find the solutions.

33

Parallel Realities

I explored past life regression for several years, sometimes three times a week. I have been into hundreds of my past lives. I realize now that they are not really past. They are only past in the way in which we perceive them in a linear manner. Really, these lives are happening now. It's easy to shift spaces or realities and connect with other versions of ourselves.

I remember the first past life I was ever taken into. I will share the story because it explains how this can work. I used to have these horrible visions, thoughts and feelings when I couldn't get in contact with my wife. When I phoned and she didn't answer I would think something terrible had happened and I would call fifteen times in a row. I would have visions of someone breaking into our house and harming my wife and children. These are not the sort of images you want every time you call a loved one and they don't answer.

When I explained this to the human being that was guiding me through my past lives she said, "*Would you like to go and have a look and see what is causing this?*" So we did. We stepped through into the Saxon era and I was on a boat with all of the other men from our village/tribe; not sure exactly what you would call it. We were packing up the boats and were leaving our reservation/village/camp and moving on.

All of the women were back at camp with the children and some men on horses rode in and slaughtered most of them. My wife and children were trampled on and had their throats cut. The men couldn't get back in time to save them. So, whilst I was away, my family were murdered.

I was instructed by my guide and teacher to go and speak to him (this aspect of my soul) and let him know that I am a future progression of his soul and that my wife and children are OK now. I gave him a cuddle and brought his light in with mine. Since that day I have never had those thoughts or vivid images.

I journeyed into many parallel realities and if you want to hear the stories then please read my book, *Into the Light.* The ability to step through dimensions and into realities is very useful when facilitating the healing of another human being. You can cross through spaces, change realities and create a scenario that manifests in the physical reality now.

It can be across space in this lifetime and others. It's all now. Your five-year-old version of you is living and playing somewhere. So is the version of you that is ten years in front. Everything can be accessed now.

A lovely lady, with stage-three cancer contacted me. Together we journeyed back through her life, connecting with different versions of herself. When we found a version that felt disconnected, we simply reconnected using love. I asked her to open her heart chakra and connect with the other version of her. We went all the way through her life until she was four years old. At four years old it was very traumatic. Once the connection was made and that little version of this beautiful human being felt loved, the cancer vanished.

I could see it in the hologram in my mind's eye; it wasn't there anymore. When this lady went back to the doctors and got the all clear she was amazed, and so were the doctors. It had completely gone.

I also find that you can send a dis-ease back to where it came from. It doesn't necessarily have to be from earlier in your life. It could be from another space or reality. So, if you ask to bring up the hologram of the human being you are facilitating the healing of, in the space that contains the dis-ease, you will see them or feel them. Once you do you can send the dis-ease or so-called problem, whatever that may be, through space to the other reality.

A really simple way to do this is as follows: In the hologram see a shape. You can pick any shape. For example, a square. You can visualize this square anywhere in the body. Once you have done this you must know that this square contains all of the emotional or karmic stuff that triggered the disease. See the square fill up with it. Place one hand on the square. Next, with your other hand feel a point in space away from the client's body, in empty space. Move your hand around slowly until it tingles/vibrates or you start to feel a pulling sensation.

Once you have found this spot, stop. Now, with your mind see this square travel out of the hologram, through space to the hand out in space and once it gets there see it explode into white light. It's that simple.

Now, I have noticed when you do this that you eliminate the dis-ease in both realities. It somehow cancels both of them out so don't ever think that you are passing the dis-ease to another version of you in another reality. You are actually doing both versions a massive favour.

When you are facilitating the healing of someone you may have to try more than one of the ways I have shared in this book. It's important to drop into the healing zone and feel, see and trust. Whatever comes into your consciousness will somehow be useful. It may not make sense but it will help you. Your right brain picks up information that your left brain cannot organize.

If you want a quick way to experience this go to the jungle in Brazil and drink Ayahuasca. It's the bark of a tree mixed with the flowers of another. It opens your Corpus Callosum completely and you see the truth. You see life for what it really is. You will look at your leg and see shapes and symbols (geometry) not flesh.

I looked down at my body and saw nothing. It was not there. I was pure consciousness hovering through space. You clearly see into the space between spaces and get the chance to communicate with other beings there. You will see, with your physical eyes that the world is one unified field of love. This is how I see the world when I drop down into the healing zone. Patterns of light, shapes, symbols and a multitude of variables are available. All of this is contained within you too. I actually see this now without any medicinal plants but it's a great way to see what is our potential, quickly.

When facilitating the healing of another human being, once you drop into your heart you can ask to be taken back to the trigger or root cause of the issue that is causing the symptom. Often it may not be in childhood but in a different time space, say two thousand years ago. Now you may not be able to see this reality or lifetime and that is OK. Some people see less than others. Sometimes I see the human being's past life or parallel reality clearly, other times I don't.

Another way that works well is this. Place two hands on your client's hologram, wherever you feel drawn to. Next, set your intention to go back to the place/space/time or root cause/trigger of this particular issue. Then feel as you drift back, in your mind through time and space. Once you stop, look around that space for a human being. If you see one great. If you don't, create one. Just visualize a human being. Man or woman it doesn't matter. If you can't visualize a man or woman, then create an object. It can be anything. Next, you must know that this object/human being represents the past life or root cause of the particular ailment of the client you are healing.

Once you have entangled the two, surround the object or human (the one you created or visualized) in a purple/violet flame and see them transmute into white light or particles and all that is unnecessary disappear. Once you have done that see a tube appear. I normally see a light tube, a little like a laser, it comes in different colours. Trust the colour that comes. It connects the client to the object or human you visualized or created and that is now white light or particles, however you visualized it.

Once connected I see the light from the past life/parallel reality get swallowed up into the tube of light, travel all the way back through time and space and into the human being I am facilitating the healing of. This works. Somehow it shifts the pattern that was causing the problem.

All of these tools are your healing tools. Sometimes you may have to select two or three. Sometimes you can take your target out in one go. Just move and flow in your healing environment. Be in your heart and trust. TRUST, TRUST, TRUST.

34

Shadow Parasites

When you read a lot of books on healing or the esoteric arts most people share their views on the good, the light side of the force so to speak. But what about the darker side? It's easy to brush it under the carpet and pay no attention to it. And a lot of people do this. There are fourth-dimensional entities that feed off of human fear. Fear is their food source. People enter into karmic contracts with Shadow Parasites in a time of desperation. They come in many different forms and will ruin your life, if you let them.

I've seen marriages break up, people attempting suicide and others completely taken over, being used as a host. A little like the film, Alien with Sigourney Weaver. This is no film however. This is as real as you reading the words on this page. I'm going to be honest with you. I was going to leave this out of this book. I was going to focus on the light; however, I am adding this section in after attending two spiritual exhibitions at the weekend where, on each of the days I performed two modern-day exorcisms.

No, I wasn't waving a cross, shouting Holy Scriptures and levitating the human being's body in the air but I did remove several Shadow Parasites from inside these two humans. It just reinforced for me the importance of sharing this information.

The first lady knew when these things had entered her. She was at a spiritual development course three years earlier. The man running the course had taken them through a meditation. These things had entered her there and then. Now you can't blame the guy running the course because Jennifer, the lady who came to my stand, must have on some level invited them in.

What the guy running the course could have done is created a space (protected it) so that nothing could have entered the workshop space, on any level/dimension. Or explained to everyone that this is how you can ensure these things don't enter your space. Because sometimes – even if you protect the space – ones that are inside the human, can still enter. Some hang onto the outside and those ones will not get into a protected space. They will wait at the door.

A great way to protect your personal space is to put yourself in a pyramid of light or an Octahedron, an eight-sided shape. It looks like two pyramids stuck to each other back to back. Each one of us actually has an Octahedron as a part of our extended human Light Body Field (we will be delving deep into that in the next Star Magic book) and how you can fully activate that.

A great way to protect the room space you are in is to cover each wall in four triangles. Flat sides at the edge, and the points folding into the centre to meet in the middle. You then seal the wall in light and cover each wall in the room. Nothing will get through a triangle. It's the most powerful shape for protection.

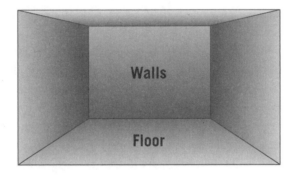

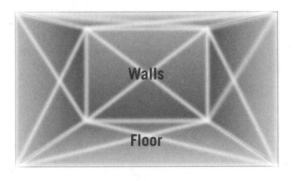

53. Protected walls

Danger itself is very real but fear is a choice. You must realize that Shadow Parasites exist but you should never fear them. On your spiritual journey they may try and step in and manipulate you, in some way, shape or form. They are great shapeshifters. They can morph into anything, often angels. You have to question what you see in the spirit world. If you see an angelic-looking being then cover it in white light. Hold it in the white light. If it remains, it's good. If it runs or moves from your space you know it's not so good. Now, sometimes, even in white light they will stay and so you must hold that space and increase the intensity of the white light to be sure.

It's important to remember that Shadow Parasites are lost. They are not evil, even though they don't do very nice things, like take over your human body. These things themselves live in fear. They want nothing more than to return to the light. They just don't know it. They are still a part of nature, just like you and I. It's simply a different vibrational frequency but natural just the same. They are an aspect of you.

There are nine musical notes and the fifth of those is of a lower vibration, one that takes you out of your heart centre. It's what the majority of Western music is based on. So when you listen to the latest pop songs you are being taken away from love and towards disharmony and fear. Coincidence? Certain music is being used as a weapon of mass destruction. Either way it's important to realize that as these vibrations are naturally occurring they are a part of nature.

So these beings that reside in this world that feed off of our fear, are a part of nature. It's a part of the grand design. We must be aware of them and remember how to play the game. It's just a game of separation in this dualistic human YOU-Niverse. Once you know the rules the game is a cinch.

Remember everything, at first, was created by love. There are some exceptions, entities created in laboratories by some Governments and secret covert operations (military) but that is a whole other story and not for this book either.

The first time I ever came across a Shadow Parasite inside a human being was back in 2006. Some friends and I went to a house in Basingstoke, England. A man was giving a talk on 2012 and the end of the Mayan calendar. I was new to all this spiritual "stuff" and very curious. Two friends and I drove down there. We pulled up to a dated bungalow and went inside. We knew no one there. Most of the people sitting there were a lot older than us. We were in our mid-twenties and they were in their fifties and sixties. My friend found out about this talk on the Internet, when he was googling "2012".

We sat there listening to this guy: I will call him Tony. I asked him a question, which he must have taken a little personal. I was not attacking him but my question, in a way, contradicted what he was saying. I was just curious.

He stopped and looked at me. He held my stare and I saw his face change. His human face disappeared and a Reptilian face came through. It was green and, well, just looked like a lizard.

In my mind I was thinking, *"What the fuck, is this really happening?"* I was seeing this with my physical eyes not with my mind's eye. On the outside I stayed cool as a cucumber but on the inside I was on fire. After several seconds his face morphed back into his human form and he carried on talking. We stayed for the rest of the evening and then drove home.

My friend dropped me off and I went and took a shower. I didn't speak to my friend until the next morning but this is what happened when he got home. He got out of his car and he said he felt someone behind him breathing down his neck. When he turned there was no one there.

As I said, when I arrived home I took a shower. I was showering away and I saw this picture of a man in my head. I shook my head but he wouldn't go. He said, *"My name is James. I'm here to protect you. That man you met earlier is trying to play mind games with you. He is attacking you psychically."*

James was an old man and he was the first of my Light Beings, Guides, Angels, whatever you want to call them that I met. I had a conversation with him in the shower. After I got changed I went downstairs, lay on the sofa and spoke with James for over an hour. It was incredible. It was just like speaking to another human being in my living room. James was the first of my guides and has been there ever since. He's honest and will always tell you straight. He gives me the very best advice.

Anyway, back to this lady at the exhibition. She came and sat in a chair where I was facilitating healing and told me what was happening. Before I even started working, this Shadow Parasite (there were two actually inside her) started talking. It was making her scratch her own face and saying disgusting nasty things. It certainly didn't like me being there, or her being in my presence. It was calling me evil. Her voice sounded completely different.

When you have to face a situation like this you don't want to go into battle. Even though it can seem like these things are horrible, remember they originated from the same energy source as you did: love. They have simply gotten lost on their journey. I'm not, in this book going to go into the history of how these entities get lost. You can read about that in my book *The Vortex of Consciousness*, if you wish to know the truth.

The way to clear someone from Shadow Parasites is to coax them out. Talk to them, negotiate with them, show them the light and guide them to it. You may have to be a little stern with them but they will come. The first

Shadow Parasite in this lady was very dark. It had black scales and a tail and huge claws. Remember, I have no right to rip this thing out. The host, in this case the lady in my chair had made a contract, albeit subconsciously, with this being and who am I to interfere with this?

I managed to lead the first one down a tunnel I created, with the help of Archangel Michael, back to the light. Once these things get to the light they love it. It's just getting them there that is the issue. Sometimes it's easy and other times it's not.

The second one of these beings I needed a little help with. It was determined, even more so than the other one, to stay. I brought the lady out of the tranced state I had her in and told her she would need to work with me on this one and that I would guide her. As I was guiding her, sharing the same vision with her, she was telling it (the shadow parasite), in no uncertain terms that it no longer had a place inside her mind, body or soul. It was no longer welcome and must leave, NOW!

I created a pyramid (completely surrounding her) in the ether and a tunnel leading from this lady's throat and into the pyramid. I created the pyramid so this parasite could not escape once it had left her body. I often go in through the navel to clear Shadow Parasites but this time the throat is what I was guided to. I coaxed this thing, again, along with Archangel Michael's help and we eventually, after forty-five minutes, led it down the corridor and into the tunnel. It went berserk once in the pyramid but then Michael took it through a door and back to the spirit world. It was extremely happy once it was back.

The lady in my chair morphed back into her human form and her face changed. She looked ten years younger and she looked and felt light and vibrant. It's important to know that it's not all sunshine and rainbows when doing this work. On the other hand, it's exciting and there is never anything to fear.

Just another situation to deal with. Stay calm, don't go into battle, and talk with these things. If you're ever removing them at distance, it's important to protect your own space and that of your clients. You don't want them wandering back into the ether and you certainly don't want them wandering around your home or workspace. Do the job properly. Danger is real. Fear is a choice. Each time you remove a shadow parasite it's different. No situation is ever the same. Just like facilitating a normal healing session. Work with what the YOU-Niverse presents to you.

When working at distance I will put my client and my space in two crystal octahedrons. I will then put a black tourmaline pyramid in empty space away from my healing space. I will bounce my energy into the black tourmaline pyramid. I then bounce into an inverted smokey quartz pyramid. I do the work from there and then once it's done bounce back through this structure, blowing it up behind me. This is how you should work when getting started. Once you know you have cleared a number of Shadow Parasites you will not need this structure. For now, use it though. I also use similar structures when I am remote viewing certain protected targets so as not to be tracked back to my location if I get picked up.

I know that once you become light enough in your vibration Shadow Parasites will leave you alone. They give up. It's like they say OK, fair dues, this guy is so far into the light now let's prey on easier targets. Journey in, do the inner work, be in the light and you will never have any issues. It's just good to be aware of this side of life or this side of the spirit world.

And the thing is, I don't like to use the word "side" because it implies duality and we are one. So please, see through the veil of illusions and realize that love is the remedy in all situations. Love will coax Shadow Parasites back to light and love will create a healing environment to morph dis-ease into perfect health. Remember, just like the Shadow Parasites, dis-ease is an illusion. All there is, is love.

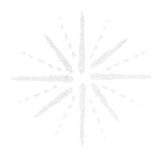

PART 5

35

Real Nutrition

If you want to be the healthiest and very best version of you it is important to ensure that the right foods and liquids pass your lips. I worked with athletes for several years in my gym in New Zealand, so I know a thing or two about nutrition. I'm not suggesting I am an expert in this field but I do know what works and what doesn't. I am also looking at nutrition in a different light these days. Before it was about athletic performance and now nutrition is a tool to aid me on my spiritual journey.

It's important to have a balanced nutritional way (programme/diet), between Light, water and food. Eventually you can cut the food element right back and bring more Light into your nutritional way. I will say "way" because I don't like the word "programme" or "plan". Feels too rigid to me. If you feel like something different today than you did yesterday, then listen to your body. There is no right or wrong method to bring more Light into your nutritional "way" as we are all unique human beings and are following our path, so based on the suggestions I shared earlier, in the book, you will have to play about with this, make some subtle changes and see what works best for you.

When it comes to nutrition the first thing I do when I wake every morning is drink a cup of my own urine. Urine therapy has been used for a long time. If you want to know more about urine therapy and the detailed benefits of urine, read this book, *The Perfect Medicine* by Martha Christy. Urine is the only liquid on this planet that contains all of the information on your own body. It is full of goodness. Uric Acid (urine) is not a waste product containing all of the "stuff" your body doesn't want. It contains all of the "stuff" your body does want but is in abundant supply. Drinking it will do you wonders.

It actually tastes OK too, a little interesting at first… and after a week or two of drinking it every day, it starts to become enjoyable. I look forward to mine each morning as strange as that may sound.

Meditation is next on my morning agenda. The silence mixed with the oxygen is very healthy. Breathing deep into your cells has so many benefits.

It is a chance for you to detox too. When you breathe deeply, you really fire up your Lymphatic system, which is responsible for sucking out all the dead blood proteins and other waste products that your body doesn't need.

Next is a large glass of juice. Vegetables and fruits. Plenty of greens in this one. Alkalizing the body is important. I won't eat or drink anything but vegetable or fruit juice up until Midday. 80% vegetables and 20% fruit is a great combination. Mostly green.

Lunch is whatever I feel like. A large salad with a mixture of colours. A variety of raw nuts. Pulses, Quinoa. I occasionally eat eggs and the odd piece of fish if my body craves it. Remember you have to listen to your body. I will never eat canned fish. It has to be fresh. I never eat chicken, beef, turkey, lamb or pork. I haven't done for a few years now. Occasionally I may have a little brown rice but not often.

I drink a lot of water. I regularly drink water throughout the day and will not wait until I am thirsty. I drink it consistently. Remember we are 75%-80% water. Our bones and muscles are 50% water, our skin is 50% water and our brain is 74% water. Our organs are pretty much all water too. In fact, we are water, space and a little bit of something very inconsequential. Water is actually liquid crystal. You can change its molecular structure with love. Drink plenty of it and don't wait until you are thirsty before you do. By then you are already dehydrated. Love or bless your water before you drink it.

Everything that I have mentioned here is pretty much what passes my lips. It may not sound like much if you're used to eating the spectrum of packaged foods on the supermarket shelves, but once you get creative, you can make hundreds or so different salads – I never get bored eating this way.

I don't eat too much in the evening. Maybe some vegetables, a green salad, an avocado with some squeezed lemon over the top of it. Just something small. I drink cups of herbal tea in the evening and more water. I very rarely drink alcohol. It doesn't do anything for me. Just makes me feel shit the next day. I sometimes get the odd craving to go out clubbing or to a pub, but whenever I have succumbed to the temptation, I just stand there thinking what a load of bollocks.

It is just a future thought of something exciting and fun, which turned out to be an anti-climax. I don't know whether it's because I partied so hard when I was younger, that maybe, now, it just seems so tame and uninteresting or maybe I just prefer to be in a park, sat under a tree meditating – where I get so much enjoyment, journeying into infinite space, and exploring the beauty of our multi-dimensional cosmic YOU-Niverse.

So nutrition is simple. Eat what comes out of the Earth. Don't cook in high temperatures. You will kill the food the farmers took an entire season to grow. Get your food locally. If you live in New Zealand don't buy grapes from Brazil. Let them eat their grapes; you can eat your own. Let's look after our planet.

If I haven't mentioned the foods that you eat, above, it's for a very good reason. Nourish the house of your soul in this lifetime. Care for it and it will give you so much in return. You really are a natural being, just like a tree. You need water, oxygen and light. Eventually we will not need food. It keeps us locked in this 3D reality.

36

Star Magic Codes of Consciousness – The Secret Recipe

Here is the dialogue between me, and a little voice, one day:

Voice: "Jerry, we are all binary code."
Me: "What do you mean we are all binary code?"
Voice: "We are all binary code."
Me: "Tell me what you mean."
Voice: "Your brain is a biological computer. It can be programmed and re-programmed."
Me: "How?"
Voice: "I am going to make it even easier for you to heal. Much faster and more effective."
Me: "Excellent. Show me."
Voice: "You are consciousness and whatever consciousness decides and intends will take place."
Me: "What do you mean?"
Voice: "Codes."
Me: "What codes."
Voice: "Remote viewing is accessed through codes."
Me: "Please explain."

At this point I had a clear vision enter my consciousness of what this all meant. A deep knowing came over me. I am going to explain this to you before I talk about these codes to give you a clearer understanding of what I am referring to.

In the military they use what is known as remote viewing. It allows a human being or several human beings, (remote viewers from the military in this case), to spy on another human being, several human beings or a location. With practise everyone can do this. Some people, are however, more natural than others.

Let's take a target for example. Let's use our good old buddy Saddam Hussein, God bless his soul. After all, it took a courageous soul to choose to

195

come into that life and incarnate as Saddam, knowing what was in store, but that's a story, for another time. So, if the military wanted to track Saddam Hussain they would allocate him a code – a sequence of numbers or letters or numbers and letters. They would infuse, into consciousness, the ether, the invisible intelligence, a connection between Saddam Hussain and this code or sequence of numbers and letters, based on their own perception.

Remember consciousness is intelligent and you heard what the voice said to me:

You are consciousness and whatever consciousness decides and intends will take place.

So those that want to spy on Saddam infuse this code into consciousness and connect it to the target, through their intention. The remote viewer is then told to go and view this target during their next operation. So he or she does that. They lower their heart rate, enter an altered state of consciousness, and think and feel that code. That code, which has been linked to its target, through consciousness, which is in all places at all times, takes the remote viewer to the location of this target, wherever it may be on the planet; there are no boundaries. Everything, everywhere can be accessed now.

How do I know all of this? Well firstly I have been involved in several remote-viewing incidents, and had everything I have seen confirmed by the so-called corporate powers that be. I have also "remote viewed" the remote viewers myself and seen them at work. We really do have the capabilities to be anywhere at any time.

This intelligence that created the YOU-Niverse, us, you, me, all things, is alive – it feels, it thinks, it's aware. It's also, in a way like a piece of Play-Doh. You can mould it, shape it and influence it. That is what the military does. They influence this intelligence and link targets to codes. The reason it's so easy is because we are all this intelligence. We are all consciousness. It is one continuous field of light. The light is information as I have already explained. Everything can be manipulated. In this case, the military may be using it for ill-gotten gains, but who am I to judge. Everything has its place in the YOU-Niverse.

So, back to Star Magic Codes of Consciousness. Just in the same way the military link a target to a code, I can link a feeling or a state of being, or a state of health, to a code. For example, The Star Magic Code of Consciousness for Perfect Health is 0632. The Star Magic Code of Consciousness for Calmness is 11, 11, 1. The Star Magic Code of Consciousness for Confidence is 2391. Each of these codes create a Healing Frequency (HF) as the codes, in essence, are written into the frequency.

HF 1 = Self Love
HF 2 = Perfect Health
HF 3 = Unity/Oneness
HF 4 = Awareness
HF 5 = Calmness
HF 6 = Confidence
HF 7 = Abundance
HF 8 = Willpower
HF 9 = Energy

These next 6 Healing Frequencies bring in very high-vibrational healing codes. To know when to use them will come with practise. It will just happen. You will get an inner knowing and will just simply find yourself infusing them into another human being's holographic biological computer.

HF 10 = Crystal Light/Energy
HF 11 = Angel Light/Energy
HF 12 = Diamond Light/Energy
HF 13 = Star Light/ Energy
HF 14 = Dragon Light/Energy
HF 15 = Dolphin Light/Energy
HF 16 = 13th Stone of Atlantis (Containing the codes of all other 12 stones too.)

Now, your brain is a biological computer. It's been programmed for thousands of years. Whether a programme benefits you or not – it can be re-written. If you are an unconfident human being I can re-write that programme. I can uninstall the original software that has conditioned you to be this way, and install a new and empowering programme that has you booming with confidence then.

Think about it. Your eyes see things around you. Your ears hear things in your world. This information is then filtered, severely, and you see and hear based on your programming. This is why they call a television programme, a programme. Because the viewer is being programmed. It's staring humanity in the face, yet, because of the collective programme, we go along with it. We are told what to wear, what to say, where to go on holiday, how to feel etc., etc. This has been going on for centuries in different forms. The result has been the same; it's only the method that has varied.

I have an array of Star Magic Codes of Consciousness that have re-written many a programme. They create freedom. I am not re-writing the programme with another structured programme, one with boundaries, designed to manipulate and control. I am uninstalling an unsuitable or limiting programme and installing a flexible one that has room for expansion and growth. It's not limited in any way, shape or form.

Of course, the human being in question, once I have created freedom for them, could, quite easily be re-programmed if they were to re-engage with the original system that had enslaved their mind. Here's where it gets interesting. Each Star Magic Code of Consciousness is designed to create a heightened level of awareness. So each human being will live in a place of tranquillity and space. They will see the world completely differently and so will see any signs of manipulation, long before it comes into their personal space.

When I install Star Magic Codes of Consciousness I have a recipe to follow that works wonders.

STEP 1: Using an inverted pyramid as my USB stick I create that image in my hand or in my mind.

STEP 2: I infuse the inverted pyramid with the best frequency.

STEP 3: Repeat this following passage. This is where I engage my intention.

> HF 6 is the Star Magic fully downloadable Consciousness Code for Confidence. I install this Light with creative Love and harmonious intelligence. I place this code within your individual holographic bio-computer now, to be used for mental, physical, emotional and spiritual growth. Let the light flow.

At this point these symbols would start to flow inside of my body. They will be gold in colour as though they are created by Star Dust (our original nature). That is the best way I can describe it. They will flow, in abundance, out through my body, into the inverted pyramid I am holding in my hand and then I place my USB into the head of the client receiving the healing. In through the top of their holographic blueprint.

If I am using these codes in a group-healing environment I will replace *"individual holographic bio-computer"* with *"group holographic bio-computer"*. Intention is everything.

We have a chance, now, with Star Magic, to seriously enhance life on planet Earth. We can re-write thousands of years of conditioning. We can do it quickly, efficiently and en masse. That is why my mission is to hold huge healing gatherings, where I can infuse everyone's consciousness with Star Magic. Imagine, fifty or one hundred thousand people, all in one venue. Imagine that energy, the love, the consciousness, the light, all in harmony. Imagine what would happen if we sent that love to a war zone.

Soldiers would instantaneously put down their weapons and walk from the battlefield. They are human too, and when it comes to the crunch, they will have an instant awakening, as the love pours from their soul. Star Magic is the most powerful, the fastest and most effective healing modality on this planet. It's Soul Technology. Are you ready to make my mission your mission too? Our Mission!

When I hold workshops, we have been known to blow out the power in the surrounding area when we send out our healing energies. Power surges shut down everything electrical; alarms sound on houses and cars, TVs stop working, hairdryers blow up and this is only from a small group.

Compare that to one hundred thousand and we will see immense shifts in consciousness. Star Magic is the key to a better world. Star Magic is the key to human freedom.

37

Codes and Realities – Serious Fire Power

You can flip/switch between dimensions and also create alternative realities in your mind, which can and will manifest, through your intention, observation and quantum entanglement in the physical world, now. We have discussed this already. Now, when you combine this idea with Star Magic Codes of Consciousness things get really exciting. This is where we unleash serious firepower.

The best way for me to describe this is to give you an example of how it can work. I was running a practise one day in Birmingham. I travel up there and run this practise every eight weeks. I really enjoy doing it. A lady came into see me. I placed my hands on her body and she collapsed backwards. I lowered her gently onto the floor. As she lay there I saw, in my mind's eye, this lady stuck in mud.

I created a platform in my mind and picked her up and put her on that platform. The platform tilted and she fell back into the mud. I then widened and lengthened the platform and put her back up on it. Once she was on it this time she started running. She had a great big smile on her face and was running and running. I then saw a woodland or kind of jungle environment. It was filling with water. It may sound strange but I knew I had to pull the plug, just like in the bath. So I found the plug and pulled it out. The water ran from the woodland/jungle and down the plughole.

Once I had created this new reality for this lady, whatever that actually was, I combined the new reality with a Star Magic Code of Consciousness. I literally put the information from the vision into a piece of light and created a code. I then installed that code into the lady's biological computer.

The lady was snoring really loudly throughout this process and once the code was installed, she suddenly stopped and opened her eyes, looking a little disorientated. When she came to I explained what had happened. She told me she felt like she is swamped in life and that things are getting on top of her. That she has taken too much on and feels that she cannot move at the pace she wants to. Like she is stuck in the mud. This lady, three months on, has given up several jobs she had, stopped going to college and started following her passion, which was to heal. She now has a successful healing business and is very happy.

To put a piece of reality into a code all you have to do is see a spectrum of light. Any colour. Orange seems to work for me. I see the vision/reality I created with my imagination start to flow like water into the spectrum of light until there is no vision left. I know it's all in the light. Once it is in the light I can then take the light code and infuse it into the human being's biological computer.

We can create codes and realities for all situations. The possibilities are infinite. They are only limited to your perception and view of reality. Know that all things are so and all things will be so and if they are not you can create them, now.

When I look at the spectrum of light I will see it as a shape. It could be a square or a triangle or any shape for that matter. Something that works really well is to see the light as a memory stick. One you would put into a computer. You then put the reality into the memory stick and then place the memory stick into the top of the human being's head. Once the download has taken place you can take it out and put it away in your pocket, ready for next time.

When you are shifting realities around, or resetting realities, which is often the case it's important that you are clear about what you want. Let me give you an example of a client of mine. I asked her what she would like to get out of the session and she told me to erase everything. I asked if she was sure and she said yes.

During the session I saw her in the middle of all versions of herself in this lifetime. They were in a circle. I asked them all to step forward and show their love and affection. They all stepped forward apart from one. I asked what age it was and it was her seventeen-year-old self. So I knew something would have happened at the age of seventeen that was blocking her. At this point a huge download of light came through me and into this lovely human being and I saw the seventeen-year-old self move towards her with an open heart.

When the session was over twenty-five minutes later I asked what happened at the age of seventeen and she explained that she got married at seventeen and she didn't want to. She did it for security and has not been living an authentic life since. Now, fast-forward thirty-six hours and everything went into overdrive. Remember, she asked to erase everything.

She was at work on Monday morning and a customer walked in, an elderly gentleman and asked when she was leaving her job. At this point she was unaware that she was. There had been no discussions and she had no plans to. Then within the hour her boss walks in and gives her a disciplinary for missing an important deadline – a deadline that she knew nothing about. That evening her husband tells her he wants to sell the house and move on. There goes the house, the husband, the family and the job – all in one go.

Now, a lot of people would freak out at this kind of upheaval. Luckily this lady knew what she had asked for and we had discussed the possible emotional roller coaster induced by her intention. *So, the moral of the story is that you will get what you ask for.* Be sure it's what you want. *You must also trust in what happens.* Even if it doesn't make sense, know that it will, in the end, be for your greatest growth as a spiritual being living this human experience.

I want to share with you one more story. When you are aware, as this human being was, you can see the beauty in all things. This is a letter I received one day:

Dear Jerry,

Please find enclosed my original letter and cheque from speaking to you last Monday. I am sorry about the deal but I ended up in hospital that day.

The amazing thing was that previously I had started doing your meditations and on the following Monday evening I mistakenly gargled with surgical spirit and swallowed some and was admitted to hospital. After being checked over I was fine. But here is the astonishing part.

They picked up a heart problem I didn't know I had and informed me if I hadn't gone into hospital that night I would have had a stroke or a heart attack. I really believe some divine intervention occurred.

I thank you so much as I feel through your meditation videos,
I had started to connect with pure love of the Universe, thus
saving my life.
Once again, thank you so much Jerry for extending your love
and knowledge to us all. I can't wait to see what happens next.
With much love and gratitude,

Val

This is a reality shift. The opening of Val's heart and connection to spirit has changed her perception. Her reality has shifted and now she sees the beauty in all that is, the guidance in every happening. You see, the surgical spirit would at first seem like a terrible thing to some people but it was a blessing in disguise. When we are open, living in our hearts, trusting and following our intuition, life is a consistent stream of miracles.

Are you ready to open your eyes?

38

Advanced Star Magic Ways

Now this is where it gets fun, really interesting in fact. In your mind there is consciousness or, maybe your mind is consciousness. Or, maybe, consciousness is mind?

Anyway, consciousness runs the show. It grows your hair, makes you sweat, pumps your heart and many other wonderful things naturally occur in our bodies due to consciousness. Scientists have examined the human brain, the human body, they have monitored the fibres in the nervous system and worked out how thoughts command the nervous system, through electrical impulses, to fire in a certain way, which, in turn, will cause muscles to contract and expand, joints and bones to move and the body to do what it has been created to do.

So-called experts know which parts of the brain are related to which movements of the body and which elements of the nervous system signal other areas of the body. In a logical sense everything can be tracked and recorded, but only so far.

The brain is like a command centre; that is clear. Where scientists hit a brick wall is when they try and work out who is running the command centre. Who is the commanding officer? It seems that no one or no-thing is. But how does it all work? Consciousness – the invisible intelligence that created, and is, all life, animate and inanimate.

If consciousness is invisible, and can function without actually being connected to anything tangible, it must mean that things can be controlled and moved remotely without being touched – this we know already.

Now, when it comes to being a Star Magic Facilitator the ultimate skill-set is developed by using nothing but your heart and your observing mind. No hand movements, no touch, no visualization, no nothing. Nothing apart from knowing. So how do you facilitate the healing of others without doing anything? Well, we are human beings not human doings. Know this and you will know.

This takes knowing to a completely new level. To remember this element of Star Magic you must go deeper. You must dissolve all elements of fear, all thoughts; you must completely empty your mind and drop into your heart space. Not half and half. Not 70/30 or even 95/5. I am saying you must go all the way. To do this requires practise, dedication and a willingness to open your heart, unconditionally to all that is, to master the art of Star Magic.

There are two phases, steps, which will allow you to master the advanced art of Star Magic. Step one will make step two easier. You can go straight to step two and I have seen it done. I have also seen many frustrated people that have tried to miss out step one and go straight to step two. Trust me, step one is worth mastering first. But you make your own decision. Remember this is a disciplined, non-systematical way of knowing. The choice is yours, baby!

Step 1

Let me give you an example of how this works. Firstly, remember, we are multi-dimensional beings. You will need to open your mind to all possibilities. If there is an inkling of doubt, it won't work. So I am sat in my healing chair, in my healing room, inside my physical body.

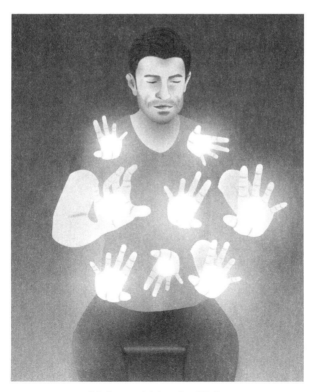

54. Jerry with hands of light

I look at the picture of the human being I am about to facilitate the healing of. I then, with my mind, see a number of arms and hands coming out from my body. All of these hands are healing the human being. There is light coming from these hands. I don't know what this light is doing specifically, apart from the fact that I know it's changing reality patterns and creating a healing environment for the human being on the receiving end.

I am not moving a muscle, yet the human being is being healed. At the same time, I can bi-locate to their location. You may want to do this to start with. Just to see what is taking place.

Step 1a

Next you can do the same thing and see your multi-dimensional selves leaving your body and standing or sitting around your client. When I facilitate healing this way, people will often say they could feel other people in the room with them.

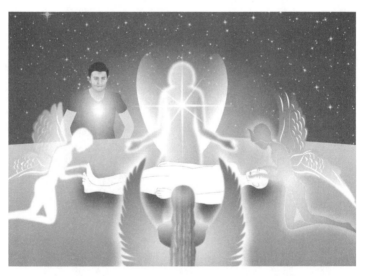

55. Multi-dimensional selves – angelic beings healing

I have pictured my multi-dimensional selves as angels. That is not always the case. You are unique and you will have to wait and see who appears when you call upon them. You will see the light flowing from their hands and see them moving around, touching different parts of the body. You are not controlling this. They know what to do. You must step out of the way, resist the eagerness to control the situation and let nature take its course.

Step 2

This is where total trust comes into play. And I mean total trust. Not 99.99999999999% trust. I mean total trust. You are going to see a client of yours and then close your eyes. Once you get the hang of this you can keep them open. You may be at that stage already. So you see your client. Then all you need to do is put your intention out:

I am going to use Star Magic to facilitate the healing of _____. I will infuse this healing with love [open your heart at this time]. I will infuse this healing with perfect health, confidence, acceptance and truth." [You can say whatever you feel you must say.]

There are no "set-in-stone" guidelines here. Next, you will ask:

Please show me something I don't know to help me facilitate the healing of this incredible human being.

This is Star Magic, baby!

Once you have set your intention know that it is taking place. Empty your mind. Be a vessel for consciousness. Do not get involved. This is where the best healings take place. Now, to start with you may find that your ego starts to try and interrupt proceedings. It may say:

This isn't working. You're not doing anything.
How can you charge people when it's not you healing?
Is this really working?
This isn't working.
Stop this at once. You have gone completely nuts.
This is your imagination running wild. Enough is enough.

Your ego will say all sorts. Liquorice allsorts. No, seriously it will throw the whole kitchen sink at you – and the kitchen, trying to make you think that this is not working or not possible. And, let's face it, it is one thing healing at a distance but it's another healing at a distance and not doing anything.

Well, remember your heart beats without you doing anything, your kidneys and liver function without you thinking about them. Your nails and your hair grow and you don't lift a finger. If this is the case, why does it seem far-fetched that you can heal without lifting a finger?

It doesn't to me. I have experienced it. It may not to you either. What needs convincing is your ego, and that my friend is something you do not want to waste your time with. What is important is for you to sink so deep into your heart, that your ego cannot play the game in this arena. The best way to sink deep into your heart is to use the dropping down exercise with the water I shared earlier. After enough practise you will be able to drop into your healing zone in a heartbeat.

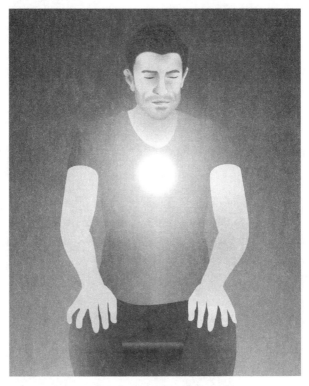

56. Opening the heart chakra

I would like to share another quick and easy (5-step) way to drop into your heart.

1. Take several long deep breaths.
2. See your heart centre as a Vortex spinning clockwise.
3. See it get faster and faster and fill with golden light.

4. Bring your awareness into your Vortex and become it.
5. Allow the Vortex to carry you wherever you wish to travel.

Your ego is comfortable in the space of your head, not in your heart. Your heart knows presence. Your ego knows past and future. Sink deep within your own heart and you will access Star Magic's true nature. By going through this book and practising the earlier ways and getting results, you will know Star Magic works. Then, gradually you will progress and start infusing Star Magic Codes of Consciousness, into your awareness. Then, when you come to this advanced way, you will naturally bring all of those other tools with you.

This is where believing and knowing truly separate themselves. I don't like to use the word separate because everything is a part of one stream of consciousness. In the realm of this advanced way, however, knowing is the only solution. As soon as you try and think, which is what believing is, a thought process that can trigger an emotional response, you create barriers. This advanced way works, only when you are pure consciousness. You are no longer a body. You are integrated with the one stream of consciousness, the one reality, the energy that is all life, Love.

You can try using this on your partner or friends, or clients that are happy for you to experiment with. You must build confidence and the best way to do that is to get results. So saddle up and get stuck in. Know that you are your own power. You are the YOU-Niverse.

As you begin to harness this absolute and total connectedness in all its glory, you will start to facilitate the healing of others, by influencing the YOU-Niversal Database with the use of your powerful, untainted, ego/fear-free intention and elevate the lives of your fellow brother and sisters. This will happen for you. There is, however, another element to this knowing...

39

Seeing – One Step Further

That element is seeing. With practise and consistent effortlessness, you will sink into this field of opportunity and possibility and create change very quickly. It will be very easy for you. The next stage is to sink into this pool of connectivity and see everything that is happening. You see, when you are taken over by spirit, by love, you can and will drift into the unified field, unaware, blissed out by the divinity of this intelligent nature, and be so wrapped up in this subatomic realm that you become oblivious to the change you are invoking in the world of the five senses.

Your mission is to see, to watch, to observe the manipulation of light, energy, patterns and realities and the change in frequency before your very eyes. Just as you would watch a television screen, you can see the wonderful world of atoms and particles at work, dancing, moving and operating at a level of super-consciousness, creating an environment whereby healing can take place.

To see this is not to visualize. To see is to observe. When you watch the manipulation machine, the television, you just sit back and interpret, you don't visualize, not in the sense that most people are used to anyway. Really your mind and the television are both two screens, screens of a different nature. The difference is the level of filtration.

When you are observing the facilitation of a healing experience, with you as the vessel and consciousness as the driver, or controller, you have, when fully open, zero filtration. When watching the television or the world go by, you are filtering the streams of light, that hit your eyes, then open up into your brain, enabling you to see a watered down version of reality.

It's still reality – just a dimmed, dull, and dismal version. When you sink into your heart and become rhythm and vibration in all its glory, a vessel that is open enough to allow source energy to facilitate the healing of another human being, you are, when you can hold the space, seeing a full version of the truth – and that is one energy source/field with zero separation.

The difference between sinking deep enough to see and sinking deeper into the state of conscious unconsciousness, is very fine. It's like that French

210

fella, Philippe Petit, who walked across a metal tightrope, a quarter of a mile above the streets of New York, in 1974, between the twin towers when the margin for error is infinitesimally small. In the same regard, it is very easy to slip from the place where you can see everything, to the place where you heal but are not aware of the knowing and cannot see.

Now it's not imperative to see. The healing will still take place but to go this far and not see is like taking a beautiful someone, of the so-called opposite sex, or maybe the same sex, out for dinner, then back to your home, or theirs, where you proceed to indulge in hours of foreplay and love making. Then just before orgasm, when you are making love with universal rhythm, as you become one, your fields of energy and your bodies become unified, you stop, pull away and don't reach that orgasmic wonderland where your merged bodies vibrate in a frenzy of oneness.

Why would you go that far and then stop? Why would you put all this effort into remembering Star Magic and not get to see the beauty and the majesty of that which you have created. It is like walking to the top of Kilimanjaro and coming straight back down before admiring the views.

So practise finding this entry point. Here you are Christ Consciousness. Here you are at one with God – You are God. You are the YOU-Niverse. In this state you transform into a subatomic blend of space, colours and fields of light. This is why you came here.

The best way to practise dropping into this state, and, at the same time maintaining your awareness, so you can see, feel and fully appreciate everything that is happening, is to get yourself a glass of water as I suggested earlier. Make sure you fill it so the water is almost level with the top of the glass. Hold the glass in two hands and place it on your lap as you sit in a chair. Start to breathe deeply and slowly. Really long deep breaths, right down to the pit of your stomach and then back out again slowly.

When I first remembered how to do this I slowed my heart rate down so much it felt like I was breathing once or twice a minute. When I actually monitored my heart rate I was around thirty beats per minute. Somewhere between twenty-five and thirty-one beats (I used a heart rate monitor) per minute, each time I did this.

As you get down to this very slow heart rate your brain waves actually slow down also. When you are in the Theta State your brain waves move at 4-7 cycles per second. This is deep meditation. The next stage is Delta, which is 0-4 cycles per second. I am not exactly sure where I am personally, when I drop into this state, but you are somewhere, I feel, just beyond Theta, crossing into Delta. Hopefully I will have the chance to measure this at some point and verify my feeling.

As you slow your breathing down, have your intention on your Third Eye and then ask to be taken to a place you know. It could be anywhere. A friend's house or another building you know. Start exploring. This is remote viewing. You want to be able to explore without spilling the water in your lap. If the glass stays full you may not have gone far enough. If it spills you have gone too far. I have found that the best way is to feel trickles of water down the side of the glass, running slowly through your fingers. This is where you are able to maintain awareness but at the same time drop down or drop into the perfect zone for remote viewing, bi-location and ultimately Star Magic.

Once you have practised with the glass of water in a basic remote viewing exercise, explore your mind and visit places you have not been to. Ask the YOU-Niverse to take you there. Pick a location, building or ask it to take you somewhere new to explore. Once you have mastered this you can try it during a healing session.

You must remember how to drop into this perfect state. It is like walking on that tightrope. The glass stays full and you have fallen off of one side. It spills totally and you have fallen off of the other side. Let it drip or tickle over the edge and you have hit the nail on the head. You are in the perfect healing zone. It's easy when you let go. Be patient with yourself.

Once you remember how to do this, healing really does become effortless. I have received phone calls from people when I have been on the move, driving, travelling etc., and the situation has been so serious that I have facilitated their healing on the move. Now, this is not something that I recommend. Facilitating the healing of someone whilst you're driving a car could be dangerous, even though I have done it many times.

I am just trying to demonstrate that when you are in the flow, and Star Magic is second nature, being a multi-dimensional being, you can allow part of you to facilitate the healing and another part of you to drive.

Also, so many healing practitioners rely on their sacred space. Why would you do that? Everywhere is sacred. I have a healing room, yes. But I also know that if I am sat on a bench in the middle of the high street and I get a phone call, that I can stop and facilitate the healing there and then.

If I couldn't do that I would be handing the power over to my healing room. It would be as though my healing room contained some of the power that was used to facilitate the healing. YOU are the power! You are the YOU-Niverse. Don't ever question this. You are magnificent.

40

As Above So Below

Do you feel the stars are up in space? Or do you feel the stars closer? They say different star constellations are billions of light years away. Does it really matter… when you're dealing with consciousness that travels at the speed of light squared or 34.2 billion miles per second. You can be pretty much anywhere in this galaxy and further out into this Universe if you wish. After all you are the YOU-Niverse.

I know that inside each one of us is every Star Constellation we know and even the ones we do not know, or should I say, remember. The reason Star Magic is so potent is because you are connecting with the frequency of the stars. You are connecting to the frequency of our intergalactic brothers and sisters of the extra-terrestrial spirit world. They are wiser than us, as a species anyway. And there are many different species out there, or on here – on Earth! They are only wiser as a species because, remember, they are consciousness too. The same as you and I. It's all love.

I regularly visit space and sit with the most incredible beings. I remember so much there. I feel at home. I feel at one, at peace. I know when I'm sat with extra-terrestrial allies that I am one of them. I'm born of the stars, a Star Seed at the core of my being. Just like you. The atoms that create your human body are the same atoms that are created from Star Dust. Star Dust comes from the explosion of Stars.

If you journey deep into the core of Earth's most prominent Star, the Sun, you will find helium and hydrogen atoms. These combine together in the depths and heat of the Star's core and create larger atoms such as Oxygen, Carbon and Nitrogen. It's the Sun's crushing gravity that pulls the smaller atoms towards its core, where they are compressed and merge, causing a thermonuclear fusion reaction thus creating larger atoms.

— CHRISTOPHE GALFARD from *The Universe Is In Your Hands*

Such a reaction cannot take place naturally on (or inside) the Earth. Our planet is too small and not dense enough, so its gravity cannot make its core reach the temperature and pressure needed to trigger one. By definition, that is the main difference between a planet and a star. Both are roughly round Cosmic objects but planets are basically small, with rocky cores that are sometimes surrounded by gas. Stars, on the other hand, can be viewed as huge thermonuclear-fusion power plants. Their gravitational energy is so big that they are forced by nature to forge matter in their hearts.

All the heavy atoms the Earth is made of, all of the atoms that are necessary for all life, atoms that your body contains, were once forged in the heart of a Star. When you breathe you inhale them. When you touch yours or somebody else's skin you are touching Star Dust.

Whilst all of this is true on one level, the sun is actually electromagnetic. When you tune in with your third eye sight or remote view the sun effectively you will see that it is electromagnetic in nature. This is important to know as the entire Universe is electromagnetic, you included. We live in an electromagnetic Universe or Torsion Universe. The sun is also a major Star Gate for extra-terrestrial races travelling into and out of our solar system. This is a completely different topic but worth sharing. The sun is available as a portal or Star Gate due to its electromagnetic nature.

Do you see how important the Stars are? Do you see how special we are? When I am creating, using Star Magic, I am connecting the light from the star constellations above with the star constellations inside your human body. Each body part mirrors a constellation. Each chakra connects with a constellation, and in some cases with more than one. I also want you to know that there are 13 months in the calendar and 13 Zodiac signs. Why have we been taught differently? Well you have to wonder what is so powerful about the number 13? Why do they say 13 is unlucky and keep you away from it? Why is Friday 13th supposed to be bad luck? Throughout history we have been lied to and manipulated.

Now I am not going to give you a history lesson in this chapter so you are going to have to take this on trust or do your own homework. I will share this though. By changing the calendar and the Zodiac signs to 12, certain so-called power structures were able to tip the masculine and feminine balance out.

This created disharmony on the planet and control through fear was easier to obtain.

Back to the constellations. The 13th star constellation in the Zodiac is Ophiuchus, otherwise known as the Snake Bearer and is the light that powers and heals the nervous system. Quite an important star to be swept under the carpet, don't you feel?

Here is a picture of the human body and the different star constellations that link into healing our physical counterpart (see also color insert).

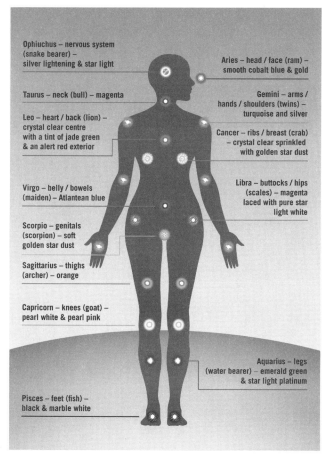

Ophiuchus – nervous system (snake bearer) – silver lightening & star light

Aries – head / face (ram) – smooth cobalt blue & gold

Taurus – neck (bull) – magenta

Gemini – arms / hands / shoulders (twins) – turquoise and silver

Leo – heart / back (lion) – crystal clear centre with a tint of jade green & an alert red exterior

Cancer – ribs / breast (crab) – crystal clear sprinkled with golden star dust

Virgo – belly / bowels (maiden) – Atlantean blue

Libra – buttocks / hips (scales) – magenta laced with pure star light white

Scorpio – genitals (scorpion) – soft golden star dust

Sagittarius – thighs (archer) – orange

Capricorn – knees (goat) – pearl white & pearl pink

Aquarius – legs (water bearer) – emerald green & star light platinum

Pisces – feet (fish) – black & marble white

57. The body with star constellations

In the above diagram you will see the Zodiac sign (its common name), the body part it is linked to and also the main colour each star uses to connect. We used to see these streams of starlight travelling through the space surrounding us and through our own bodies. But man was driven to screen this out by man's natural survival instincts. We were on the lookout for predators, driven by fear and we naturally over time, only saw what we needed to survive. Once modern technology tightened its corporate grip, we became even less aware of the beauty of our true and undivided nature.

To work with these constellations all you have to do is use your intention. You will connect with the constellation of your choice as soon as you intend it and you will see the immense rush of light flooding into that body part. You don't need to tell it what to do. It already knows. Once you open the connection with Star Light your healing abilities will go up another gear.

I am not sure how many gears there are, and I am very excited to find out. Experience this now. Play with this light. Practise on yourself or use this Soul Technology on your clients. This is super-powerful. You are Star Dust, an extra-terrestrial connected to the stars through the CNL. Start utilizing these natural and hereditary star qualities. Unleash the power now.

41

13 Chakras,
13 Star Constellations

Being in the space that we are in now, at this critical time of human and spiritual evolution it's important that we anchor ourselves into the upper dimensions, ready for ascension.

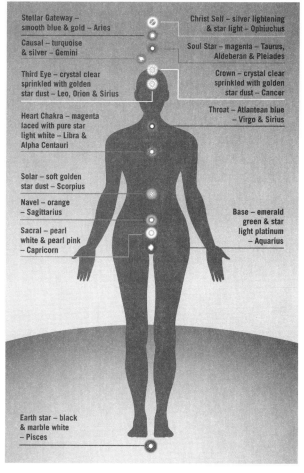

58. Chakras and zodiac signs in the body

The 13 fifth-dimensional chakras and Transmission Centres are connected to the 13 zodiac signs. This is not logical but it's the way it is. The diagram on the previous page shows the human body, the 13 fifth-dimensional chakras and the zodiac signs they relate to. It also shows the colour resonance linked to each chakra (see also color insert).

When working with these chakras all you have to do is bring the light from the zodiac into the respective chakras. You will notice that some chakras are linked to more than one zodiac sign. I suggest you play around with this. It will blow your mind – literally. Ensure you visualize the correct colours and match them with the respective chakras.

Remember that the light is intelligent and knows exactly what to do. Connecting this chakra system to the Star Constellations will raise your own vibration and the vibration of your clients 100-fold, no exaggeration. This is powerful.

You are going to know when to use this when healing. In fact, it will just happen. The more you tune into the Star Magic Frequency the further you will expand, organically. The YOU-Niverse will guide you by showing you during your healing experiences with others and when healing yourself. This element of your healing arsenal is really harnessed through experience, by playing in the Universal Database.

Once you know how to activate the chakras and body parts by using the Star Constellations this will become the main asset in your healing arsenal. Everything I have shared up until this point in the book falls in behind this knowledge. This is the cornerstone of Star Magic.

42

Human Aura

The human energy field, otherwise known as the aura, can be cleaned and cleared by using the Orion Star Constellation, otherwise known as the hunter, which carries a powerful female energy. In our auras we often carry implants given to us by external controlling forces. When you switch on your Third Eye sight you will see them. Use the light from Orion to clean and cleanse yours or anyone else's aura immediately.

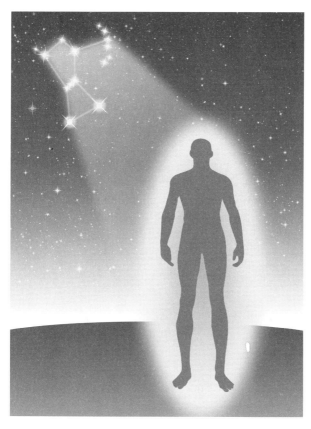

59. The human energy field with the
Orion light energy filtering in

Bring your awareness to the human being's aura and then with your intention see the light travel from Orion and connect with the aura of the client you are healing, or your own aura if you are healing yourself. Once the light hits the aura you can sit back and let it work its magic. The light coming from Orion, to clear and cleanse the aura is crystal white. Observe, play and allow.

43

Mer-ka-ba Field

Around every living organism is an energy field. This energy field surrounding people, and all sentient beings is known as the Merkaba field. In fact, the Merkaba only makes up a part of this field but a very important part it is.

Mer means special kind of light, Ka means spirit and Ba, means interpretation of reality according to the Egyptians.

In Hebrew it means vehicle and is spelt Merkabah. One thing I know from working with my Merkaba is that it holds infinite potential. The basis of your Merkaba is two Tetrahedrons superimposed over the top of each other.

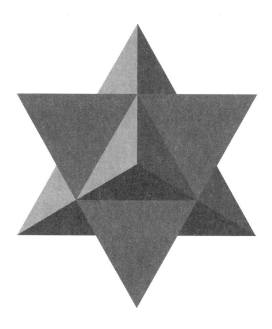

60. The Mer-ka-ba field

This Merkaba connects you with the CNL or channelled network of light I referred to earlier. It's an infinite web of beauty and power.

A human being inside their Merkaba looks like this. You will notice that, depending on whether you are male or female, the Merkaba is positioned around your body slightly differently.

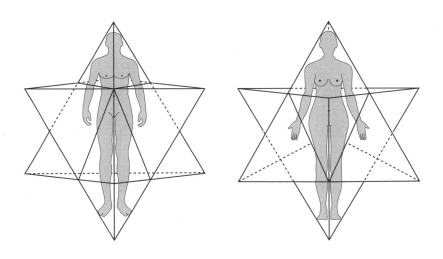

61. Man and woman inside a Merkaba

To fully activate your Merkaba you must go through your heart. You must bring your awareness into your heart and connect it with your head. You can do this with your intention. Once this link is made you can bring the star light from Sirius (male energy) into the top star tetrahedron. You then bring the star light from Orion (female) into the bottom tetrahedron.

Once this has taken place you will see that the Tetrahedrons will fill up with light. All the time you are fully in your heart. Your love is also filling up the Merkaba. Your next move is to invite the Dolphin Light/Energy in from Alpha Delphini and Beta Delphini, two stars in the Delphinius Star Constellation. Once this is done your body changes immediately. You will be lighter and will start to vibrate at a much higher frequency.

The top Tetrahedron spins clockwise as you bring the light from Sirius into it. It will get faster and faster. The bottom Tetrahedron spins anti-clockwise as you bring in the female energy from Orion. Both Tetrahedrons will spin faster and faster until they spin so fast that they look still. You will feel them spin around your body. You can activate your client's just as you can activate your own. I suggest doing this every day until they continue to spin.

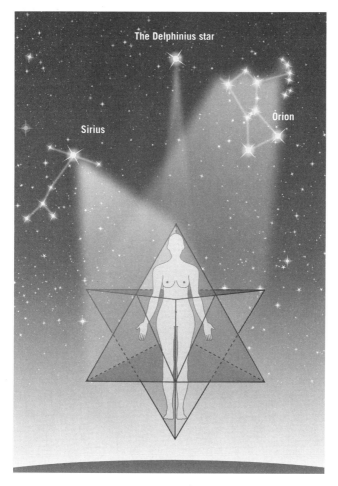

62. Star energy coming from Orion and Sirius into the two tetrahedrons, and Alpha and Beta Delphinius into the human body

If you spend 15 minutes every day bringing in these light frequencies into your Merkaba and do it every day for 21days your Merkaba will start to spin on its own accord. You will see it and feel it. Once it is spinning it will enhance and elevate every intention you have. So choose your thoughts and intentions wisely.

Once this is fully activated you will automatically connect to the Christ Consciousness Grid around the planet, which again, is created by geometry. Each human being has their own Christ Consciousness mini grid, connected to their own energy field, which then connects to the Planetary Christ Consciousness Grid. It comprises of a Pentagonal Dodecahedron and an

Icosahedron. A 12 and 20-sided shape respectively. Within this field there are a number of other geometric shapes all connected to you through atomic spin points into the channeled network of light (CNL). We don't need to go further into this right now. This is enough information for you to fully activate your human light body.

I suggest that you spend fifteen minutes every day bringing in the light energies/frequencies to activate this aspect of your miracle-creating soul machine. I also suggest spending time/space each day connecting your chakras to the Stars. This is what will activate the full potential of Star Magic. Also, with your intention connect your heart to your mind. This is mission-critical. Without that heart/mind connection you will not unleash your full human potential.

It takes dedication and discipline to be a Star Magic Facilitator.

44

Healing for Healers

Star Magic is the energy healing modality for healers. It's the Lamborghini of the healing world. It's not better, higher or more prestigious. In fact, it is subtler in a sense, and it's the subtlety that generates the power, the velocity. It's the subtlety that allows you to sink deeper into the field of love, become one with it and in turn create a harmonious, fear-free energy flow within your own body, which allows your healing abilities to heighten.

Other healing modalities are a watered down version of Star Magic. Up until this point in time, humanity – the modern version of humanity – has not been ready for a healing modality so powerful, so basic and yet so advanced. Star Magic has been around since the beginning of time. The first humans on our Earth plane knew Star Magic. It was second nature. Our extra-terrestrial allies out there in space and down here on Earth, playing amongst us, have always known this.

Over time within the human race it was forgotten, maybe it was lost on purpose. Over the centuries human beings have tried to piece the Star Magic puzzle back together again, just like Humpty Dumpty. It's been given names such as bio-energy healing, Reiki, Quantum Energy Healing and many more, and they have played their part: as perfect stepping stones, they have been great. They have served their purpose. They have bridged the gap.

To come from a place of no form of energy/light healing to Star Magic would have been, perhaps, too big a step to take. The Egyptians, the Atlanteans, our brothers and sisters living in the realm of empty space, in a lighter dimension just beyond ours, have strategically waited, patiently, for the appropriate time to enlighten the lives of this world. They have been observing and have seen too much pain and suffering, caused by the global corporations of this modern world and now feel it's time to give humanity their freedom back – to help us remember the truth.

I am the channel through which that truth is being shared. It doesn't make me special or any different; I'm simply playing out the role I knew I would play out before incarnating into this human body. I signed up for this. Now that I have remembered Star Magic I am passing it on to you; your mission is to help me spread this message. Not for my sake, but for our sakes. When I speak of "our", I am referring to our world, our beautiful big blue planet, floating in space, covered in water, ready to be healed. Star Magic can and will heal this planet. It will heal the planet by healing humanity first.

Even with more than 8 billion people on this planet, the healing can take place very quickly. Consciousness on this planet has risen very quickly in recent years. I just look at myself; I came from the streets, a drug-addict, who didn't believe in anything remotely spiritual only ten years ago. Now, my entire life has changed. If I can we all can.

Star Magic is the healing modality for healers, for one simple reason. It's going to allow all energy healing or light healing practitioners all over the world, to facilitate the healing of their clients, quickly and efficiently. What this means is that if you're an energy/light healer, you will not be seeing your clients over and over again, anymore. No! It's time to start healing your clients in one or two sessions, by causing such a reality shift that their levels of awareness heighten and they know what to do.

As an energy/light healing facilitator you will now be able to heal en masse by joining everyone's energy field together and facilitating the healing.

My mission is to heal one billion people. This will happen by you realizing your own power and becoming that power. By each facilitator on this planet, upskilling and enhancing their own ability through Star Magic, the healing will spread very quickly. If you're not an energy/light healer and are reading this book you now know how to heal yourself and others at a much higher frequency.

So now, whether you like it or not – you are an energy/light healer – but not just any energy/light healer. You have remembered Star Magic. You know how to facilitate the healing of yourself and of others. It's truly an amazing gift. A gift we all share as human beings.

If you want to become a Star Magic Facilitator you can find out more information here: *www.starmagichealing.com* I know there will be energy healing practitioners that may find it hard to step into something new; to move to another healing modality to enhance their own. Energy healers from a variety of labelled modalities come to me for healing and their ability to heal is strengthened. Why? Because Star Magic goes so deep, and connects you to an extra-terrestrial light frequency that has not been available in this manner until now.

It fully clears and unblocks the human being or healer in question and clears the pathway for extra-terrestrial light codes to upgrade your human system and create a divine, pure light body. So, in turn, enabling their own YOU-Niversal light flow to increase, enabling them to heal faster and more effectively. They naturally remember how to get out of their own way after experiencing Star Magic. You will do the same.

I have been witness to a number of energy healers who teach others and a part of the deal is that you don't tell anyone how you did it. It's like a cult, a lot of secrecy. How can something like this be a secret? If you have information, share it. I am sharing this information so you can use it – not so you lock it away and not tell anyone about it. Even one of my own family went on a Reiki course. When I asked if I could look at the material I was told no, I'm not allowed to show anyone. I almost fell off my chair. This information is available in the library.

Now Star Magic will be available in the library. It's incredible. The world is now going to be healed. The human population is ready to be uplifted to new and incredible heights. We are going to revolutionize the medical world. Elements of the medical world are using energy healing already. Now we can enhance what they are doing. Western medicine will, in the not too distant future, work with Star Magic. It will have to. Star Magic is going to create a healthy global community, and so human beings will not be frequenting the doctor's surgery or the hospital anymore. They won't need too.

They will be healthy, healed and maintained, by Star Magic. There will be resistance from corporations, because money and control are involved, but that will sort itself out with time and space. Remember healthy people don't make money within the current system – unhealthy people do. As strange as it may sound a country's GDP (Gross Developed Product) is measured using some scary statistics, one of them being the amount of people with cancer. So, the more people with cancer, the higher the GDP. Crazy but true. Star Magic will put an end to all of this.

The medical world will always serve a purpose and that will be when accidents happen; emergency surgery is necessary to stop bleeding and stabilize human life. Then, Star Magic can be used to speed up the healing process (something I have done many a time) without the use of any drugs.

Moving on from there, the power of Star Magic will be able to be used in accidents, when heavy bleeding and smashed bodies are a reality. I have been shown how to correct bone structure and stop bleeding and even heal an open wound quickly. I am still remembering and practising, opening myself more and more. Once I can remember this ability, harness it and integrate it fully, I will pass it on to you and the rest of our human family.

Consciousness is rising. Awareness is heightening. The world is changing. Freedom is happening. Our lives are unfolding. Humanity is loving unconditionally once more. Are you ready to step outside of your comfort zone, deep into the forgotten "known", and embrace this magical power?

45

Dealing with Emotions

Emotions are a part of being human. They can be controlled but why would you want to? Supressing our emotions is what creates pain and suffering and ultimately dis-ease to begin with. Holding on to the natural flow of energy is to be controlling, rigid and this will show up in your body; maybe a hardness of heart. Emotions are just energy in motion after all, and it's integral that we learn to let all energy flow naturally.

If that means floods of tears, let them flow. If it means letting off some steam by screaming, then scream to your heart's content. If you feel angry, be angry. Feel every emotion fully. Then ask yourself – why am I feeling like this? Get curious about your emotions. Feel them fully, go into them and inquire.

Befriend your emotions and you will transcend any pain that caused them. Resist the emotions and the pain will not only continue but escalate. We are human and we carry the power of choice. We carry the power to choose, in each moment, what we are thinking. We are co-creators of our own YOU-Niverse. We can choose to be present, and in doing so observe ourselves being in this world.

Or we can be caught up on the dangerous thought train, basking in illusory future events that may not ever happen but haunt us in the now, or we may jump onto the slippery slide that takes us back, into the past to experience deep regret. Neither are healthy if you get lost in this chaos. However, if you can observe your own mind, thinking these thoughts, you are on the path of freedom.

Freedom is being. Enslavement is doing. It's great to take action and create your world, your YOU-Niverse, but that action must come from a place of stillness. You must take action because you were spiritually inspired; guided by God, the omnipotent intelligence within, not that little voice in your head, that ego of yours, driving you forward through fear.

Centuries of human conditioning lies within our DNA – on a cellular level we carry information, knowledge and wisdom. We also carry the torment of every soul that has ever graced this planet. There is a tiny part of everything that ever was, everything that is, and everything that ever will be, inside each and every one of us. When you go into it, this can be the only way. When your human body decays at the end of this life, your energy source moves on. It blends back into this intelligent YOU-Niverse.

There are not really any souls. As I have said, we are one living field of energy that passes through everything. There is no separation. Using Star Magic regularly will enable you to see this field of light. You will know that the Universe is contained within every living cell in your body, thus making you the YOU-Niverse. One day you will look down at your leg and see no barriers, just a whole lot of geometrical shapes and patterns; you will see the truth.

You will be walking through the park and no longer will you see people running, dogs barking, children playing. Instead you will see patterns, outlines, energy-fields merging and blending into one continual field of energy – zero separation. You will open your Third Eye fully and see the beauty of consciousness in all its glory. You get to choose now. You get to choose always, and always, will only ever be now.

Our emotions are excellent guideposts. Signs to lead you in the direction of now. If you feel angry, sad, jealous, hurt; whatever you may be feeling, then you know that you are not aligned with your authentic nature. You have fallen away from the now – not in body but in mind. You drifted forwards into the future or you slipped slowly back to the past. The more you meditate, the more you observe, the more you use Star Magic, the easier it will be to see the truth, always. Use your emotions to guide you; don't be swept away by them.

When you are healing, and we all need to heal or we would not be here in these dense bodies, in this jungle reality, living, breathing, playing and learning. We would have moved onto the next stage of our journey, wherever that may be. I feel it is somewhere, dancing in between the light and sound codes, whistling and surfing through the dimensions beyond ours, free of these meat suits where we can mix and blend and be at one with the cosmos. Using Star Magic, you will ultimately bring everything that doesn't serve you to the surface; thousands of years of human conditioning will race to freedom.

Sometimes it escapes and passes without notice (as I have already shared) and other times you experience an upheaval, you step onto an emotional roller coaster.

People ask me if I could help them through this process using Star Magic. The answer is yes I could, but would it be wise? When you are releasing this much stuck emotion it can seem like you are in a very dark place. If I were to help you out of that dark place, then what would you learn? Your mission is to observe yourself in this dark place and experience it fully. If I were to help you out, you would lose strength. The strength to soar, afterwards. The cleansing process may not be easy but it's a necessity.

An athlete endures hours and hours of pain in training. They can't just waltz into a competition and be victorious. They go through hours of cleansing, nurturing, building, developing and learning. In your time and space of cleansing, so must you experience the same. As I said, some people bypass all of this and the conditioning simply shifts – if that is you then so be it. All is perfect in the YOU-Niverse.

It's much like a caterpillar inside a chrysalis. The caterpillar is kept in darkness, not knowing when it will get out. It must sit there, patiently. As I mentioned earlier, Scientists have helped butterflies out from their chrysalis too early. Do you know what happens when they do this? The butterfly cannot fly. It is not strong enough. It hasn't experienced, learned, grown in strength and endured the training necessary, to spread its wings as a beautiful butterfly, and fly off into the summer breeze.

As the butterfly must go through this process of nature, so must you and so must your clients, if you are planning on being a Star Magic Facilitator? It's important to explain what may or may not happen before you facilitate a Star Magic Healing session. It will enable your clients to sit in their own space and observe. Star Magic is extremely powerful and it goes straight to the root cause of any blocks. It's not always an easy ride dealing with these deep-rooted traumas. So be prepared and prepare those that you are working with.

I see a beautiful world, a heavenly reality, a joyous splendour of sharing and caring. I see a world where the planet's resources have been shared equally between all men, women and children – all human beings. I see a human race that has remembered how to care for our Mother and not deplete her, selfishly, of all of her resources.

I know this to be a possible future scenario. After all, the YOU-Niverse contains all possibilities now. So what will you choose? Are you ready to remember your power? Are you ready to unleash the Star Magic within you? Are you ready to float in the wind like Star Dust?

Just like a human being releasing stuck emotions, or as I said, a caterpillar inside a chrysalis, the human race will experience change, en masse; an upheaval as we integrate the new light and sound codes, the language of light, the language of Star Magic. Enlightened souls must hold the space, continue to love unconditionally, with compassion as our brothers and sisters acclimatize to this new way of being, in this world.

Just keep this word in mind – sharing. By sharing you are letting go. To let go is to be free. To know that you own no-thing. Even your divinity is not yours. Nothing so sacred can be owned. No-thing so sacred can be contained.

Let your divinity spill out into the world for all to see – be the inspiration that this world not only needs, but craves. Be the light. Be your light.

46

Unleash Your Full Human Potential

You are not on this Earth to live your dreams. You are here to fulfil your own destiny. You are your own prophet, exploring and sharing your greatness with the world. What is needed on this planet is 8 billion leaders. Not a handful of leaders that other human beings look to for guidance, reassurance and to be helped along their path. It's dangerous to have leaders. If you feel you need a leader, then you must unleash the power of Star Magic within yourself. Once Star Magic is flowing you will know that you are the power, that you can lead yourself, to fulfil your own prophecy.

Once Star Magic is shared in schools across the world we will create a wholesome vision, a free generation of wild flowers. After all, that is what children are; they are flowers growing in a field, humans evolving in a world of formless form. We must treat each other, especially our children, like we would a rose in our garden. We water a rose and leave it to flourish. We do not water it and pray that it flowers. We do not will it to expand in the months of spring, and let out its beautiful essence, for passers-by to enjoy. It does what it wants, when it wants, all of its own accord.

Children are born with Star Magic. They are Star Seeds who understand the light and sound codes travelling through space. They know themselves. They know Star Magic. Their power is extraordinary. They know their own DNA carries the life-blood of the planet and they live with Wu Wei, flowing, vibrating in harmony, shining as they do. We can remember so much from children, so let's let them be.

Star Magic will allow you to unleash your full human potential into this world. You, whether you know this yet or not, have the power of super-man or super-woman. You are a super-human with the strength, durability, capacity to heal and live selflessly, the ability to fly, communicate telepathically, bi-locate and so much more. Work with Star Magic every day and you will develop these abilities. You will remember them.

I was in the Philippines several months ago, on a humanitarian mission. I took a team with me to help build schools, homes; we took food relief and on my travels I met an incredible human being. I want to share this story with you, below, because the only possible explanation for this feat of willpower, and endurance, was Wu Wei. Consciousness was flowing through this man; love was inspiring him from within. God was his guide.

Oliver Conde was out diving one day, catching fish to feed his family. He surfaced too fast and it caused him to have a stroke. He was completely paralysed down one side of his body. A few months later the Typhoon Haiyan rumbled through the Philippines, destroying villages in its path. Oliver lived in a small village just outside Daanbantayan, Cebu and it was completely flattened. Everyone was crying, worried, huddling under whatever shelter they could find, as the winds swept across the open ground and the rain continued to pour.

Oliver was married, and still is, with five children. He couldn't bear to see them cold, wet and hungry. So Oliver decided to build a makeshift house out of bits of wood that he found. It took him a week, with his paralyzed body, to complete this task. Oliver wasn't satisfied with what he had built; it kept his family dry but not warm. It was also too small. They had to lie across each other to sleep. When I interviewed Oliver he explained to me it was the perfect stopgap.

Oliver decided he wanted to build a bigger, sturdier house that would keep his family warm and dry, a house they could, once again, call their home. So Oliver set to work with a hammer, some old nails he'd pulled out of the debris and wood from buildings destroyed in the typhoon. Everyone else in the village stood by and watched him. They called him crazy and no one came to help.

Oliver managed to put the wooden foundations in, and the four walls, even with half of his body not functioning. When it came to the roof it was with great difficulty but he continued on his mission. His father slung some old rope around a tree and tied it around Oliver's waist. It was used as a winch to lift Oliver up onto the roof. It took more than an hour just to get him up there. No one came to help.

The rest of the people, cowering in despair, at the fate of their village, looked on, laughing at Oliver, intermittently amongst their tears, as he continued to build what everyone else said could not be done. "Why are you doing this? You are crippled! You are crazy! You don't stand a chance! The typhoon will come again and blow it back down." Day and night Oliver had to listen to these comments.

Once Oliver was up onto the roof structure he continued to work. He then needed the toilet. He had two choices. Option one: he could spend two hours getting back down and up again or, option two: do it from up top. He chose the latter. The entire village laughed at him, continued to point their fingers, cracking jokes about this crazy crippled man building a house that would only fall again. Oliver told me he just focused on his family. He was oblivious to everything. He said he could feel God inside of him guiding him, leading him. He was spiritually inspired, by some unknown force. He told me he still doesn't know to this day how he managed to get onto the roof. It was wet, the wood was as slippery as ice and his body was paralyzed down one side. "How was this possible?", was the question he asked me.

Oliver completed the house in several weeks. His family were safe, dry and warm. Oliver continues to fish. He drags his rowing boat into the sea each day to catch fish, even with his crippled body. This is a human being that lives in the now, in the moment, happy, contented, in full acceptance of all that is. He is grateful for his family and the joy they share together.

Oliver has Wu Wei. He lives in a state of spontaneous flow. He doesn't force anything. He drifts with the tide of life and is a very happy man. You cannot try and be Wu Wei just as much as you cannot try and harness the power of Star Magic. You must be it. Once Oliver Conde completed his home, the rest of the village followed suit. Within a few months the village was restored. Oliver's divinely inspired courage inspired his fellow brothers and sisters to re-create their lives.

To be free you must know there is no right or wrong in the world. Oliver Conde could have said it wasn't fair – not right. He accepted. There was no blame. When you know that there is no right or wrong, by default, there is no blame. When there is nothing or no one to blame, you are free. Forgiveness creates freedom. Acceptance of all things as they are, is liberating. By accepting and forgiving you can change the meaning of the past. You can create the space for Star Magic to flow.

By accepting yourself, fully and unconditionally, you open yourself up, into a space of infinite possibilities. You allow your true nature to flow. You become the flow. You become Star Magic. By you being you, the real deep down you, you will set into motion a state of conscious contagion. Your vibratory state will flow throughout the YOU-Niversal Database, through the field, and like a stone dropped into a pond you will affect the entire pond. A human being vibrating with such pure and harmonious flow will cause every cell throughout the entire YOU-Niverse, to vibrate in alignment with your flow.

By unleashing your full human potential, through the use of Star Magic, you will become a clear channel for pure source energy. No blocks. No-thing will stand in the way of you creating a peaceful world. You came from no-thing and you will return to no-thing. Just remember that no-thing is not nothing. You came from a formless substance, an intelligence. This intelligence created you, it is you, and flows through your YOU-Niverse, continually.

It wants to expand you, grow you, live you, love you and be you. So kick back, trust and enjoy this magical ride. Only you can possibly stand in your own way. So get out of it now. Allow the authentic you to play, like a child, running, dancing and laughing, loving, cuddling and enjoying. This is your natural state. In this vibratory state you will unlock the magic of the stars. That is where it comes from, out there, up there, in outer space, or maybe, just maybe, the stars are within you.

It's your journey. It's your human life. You were born to play large, not small. You were created to live at a level beyond extraordinary. You are light and sound, waves of energy, an infinite number of particles created from no-thing. An illusion. Your pattern is about to become so much more – you are now expanding your consciousness, and lighting up this planet. Know your power now.

Fully explore the YOU-Niverse.

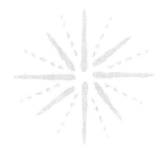

APPENDIX

Real-Life Case Stories

Here I want to share a few case stories from clients that I have had the honour of facilitating the healing of. I love you all and thank you from the bottom of my heart for giving me the incredible opportunity to work with you and your light.

Fibromyalgia

I had suffered with anxiety for a number of years. I was 42 when I was diagnosed with Fibromyalgia and was struggling to walk. I had to use a walking stick, the pain was unbearable and I put on heaps of weight. The doctors had put me on a whole lot of medication and I was pretty much rattling as I hobbled along with a stick. It was very demoralizing. My confidence had gone and I felt very depressed. I was sweating profusely, came up in an awful rash on my face and my hair started falling out.

After contacting Jerry and talking with him he agreed to help me. Not only did Jerry use Star Magic healing, he totally changed my diet. During the healing sessions I could feel the energy working inside of my body. It was a strange but nice feeling. Within four weeks I was medication free, within five weeks I was pain free and walking perfectly fine without a stick and within seven weeks I had lost more than twelve kilograms in weight. I have no confidence issues, my hair has grown back, my rash cleared up and I actually feel normal again for the first time in many many years.

When I went to see my doctor he couldn't believe his eyes. He looked at me and said, "Wow, look at you". He was so impressed at how healthy I was. I told him I had been receiving energy healing and he was very supportive.

Even now, more than a year has passed and I have been great. My life is back on track and I am so grateful. Thank you Jerry.

— KAREN

Emotional Trauma

I lost my son several years ago and have been struggling in many ways since. This event along with others in my life had caused a lot of blocks. Things were not moving in the right direction. I wasn't happy with my job, my health and most aspects of my life.

I attended one of Jerry's two-day workshops and my life has never been the same since – in a positive way. The workshop was incredible. Jerry took all of us through a series of deep meditations and group healings, which were just amazing. I was very emotional during the experience as I was connecting with my son and so much stuff came up.

The meditations and healing sessions were so deep and it felt as though years of emotional baggage from this life and previous ones had risen to the surface. After the workshop I went on an emotional roller coaster. I had never experienced anything like it. I was prepared for it though as Jerry had told me what to expect. I sat with my emotions like Jerry suggested and they passed.

My confidence grew, I started eating healthier, I lost more than a stone in weight and I decided to quit my job and trust that everything would work out. Within a week or so of leaving my job the Universe just opened everything up for me. I started to follow my passion as a therapist and was offered a position that was just right in every way. It is as though the energy at the workshop cleared the path for everything in my life to slot into place – and it has.

I am so happy and see the world completely different now. I get so much joy in the simplest of things, like a tree or a flower. I have a new lease of life and am ever so grateful to Jerry.

— DEBBIE

Trigeminal Neuralgia

A lot of dark things were happening in my life and I was suffering from a chronic condition called Trigeminal Neuralgia. I had been prescribed all sorts of medication by the doctor and it just made me worse. I felt even darker and more depressed and I was in severe pain down the side of my face.

The issues around what was happening spread into my personal life and I didn't know how much more of it all I could take. Things just spiralled out of control and I was in an extremely dark place when Jerry came into my life.

After discussing everything with Jerry we did the first healing. I could feel Jerry working throughout my body, especially around my heart. Over the course of a few weeks and two more healing sessions I felt so much better – lighter. Jerry gave me a method to come off the pharmaceutical drugs I was on and I followed it.

I came off slowly with no trouble at all. It took about eight weeks to come fully off of the drugs and I felt as though I was back to normal. Somehow Jerry raised my vibration. Each session I could feel my vibration going up. I now feel fearless, all the pain has gone and my life is better than ever.

— KERRY

Suppressed Emotions from Death of Husband

Over the years, I've been fortunate enough to receive several Distance Healings which have proved most beneficial, but have never experienced one that had such a powerful and immediate effect as I received from Jerry – which released so much of the suppressed grief I'd been carrying for almost thirty-five years since the sudden and entirely unexpected death of my first husband.

In a state of shock, I misguidedly believed – at that time – I needed to "be strong" for my two young sons, my distraught mother-in-law and my elderly parents to whom my husband was the son they'd never had.

I was so caught up in my supportive role, and busy making funeral arrangements, attending to all the practicalities of life ensuing from a sudden death etc., and having to return to work within a few days, I just couldn't find time to express my own feelings and tears, not even in bed at night, as for a long time afterwards, my youngest son slept with me – being afraid to let me out of his sight, in case I too passed on. Thereafter, as life was so demanding, and I was busy dealing with the "now", the pain of my loss became buried underneath it all.

A couple of hours after the Healing session with Jerry, I felt as though a tap had been turned on in my head, as my eyes and nose started to run uncontrollably – the unshed tears of all those years before, and then I started vomiting – releasing the unexpressed and "forgotten" feelings of grief I'd been holding on to. It was an intense, but very brief period of "activity", after which I felt physically, mentally, emotionally and spiritually at Peace. Thank you.

— CHRIS

Perthes Disease

I am thirty-eight years old, a successful hairdresser and business owner. I was feeling low on energy, a lack of creativity and felt that I needed something to give me a boost. I contacted Jerry and after talking with him I felt he could help me.

I didn't tell Jerry about my sore hips and that they were hindering me whilst stood all day cutting hair. And, that they stopped me working out properly in the gym. I just told him I was lacking in energy and creativity and wondered if he could help. When the healing was taking place I was lying down on my bed at home. My body went hot – really hot and then my legs started to lift up into the air. The soles of my feet turned inwards and touched and I was under the blanket. The blanket rose up in the air too. My legs were up for a good couple of minutes.

My arms seemed to take on a life of their own too. They rose up really slowly and I couldn't control them. They arched on the top of my head and again I had no control over this. I have tried to get into this position again, since the healing, and I can't. It's impossible.

My legs went down and I thought phew, it's finished. It was like relief running through and out of my body. Then they rose again. It was the most extraordinary experience I have ever had. Being moved around by someone or something that you cannot see, and at the same time I felt very reassured.

When I spoke to Jerry after the healing he told me that he saw me in callipers at the age of six. That is how old I was when I had Perthes Disease. He didn't know this so this shocked me. Since the healing I have had no pain in my hips and can now fully function at the gym. My energy levels have gone through the roof and my creativity is flourishing again. I am getting new

241

and inspiring ideas on how to expand and grow my business and my staff have noticed a massive difference in me.

I can't recommend Jerry enough. He has changed my life.

— ASHLEY

Cancer

I had been diagnosed with prostate cancer and had received treatments from the medical profession. It seemed to stifle it and then it got progressively worse. I was looking for something alternative, searching the Internet one day and The Facilitator popped up on Google. I contacted Jerry and felt he may be able to help.

During the healing I didn't really feel like anything was happening. I thought maybe all this distance healing was a con or a hoax. Anyway I spoke with Jerry after and decided to do another few sessions. We did seven in total. After the third session I started to feel as though things were improving. At the time I was struggling to urinate. It was coming out slowly. I felt as though I needed to go but the tumour inside me was getting in the way. Jerry also asked me to change my food intake. He wrote a plan for me asking me to add certain things in and take certain foods out from my diet. It wasn't easy but I agreed. I was prepared to do anything to be healthy again.

Within three weeks I could pee normally again. I kept thinking am I imagining this? I went back to the doctor on my next visit and my blood count was better than before. I remember looking in the mirror and thinking to myself how much better I looked. People were commenting that I looked younger. I felt it.

My blood count is now normal. The doctor's scans showed no signs of any tumours. I didn't ever tell my doctor what I had been doing apart from that I had started to eat more greens. Maybe it was a combination of the medical treatment and the Star Magic from Jerry.

Maybe it was just the Star Magic. We will never know for sure but one thing I am certain about is Jerry played a huge role in me getting my life back. He also supported me mentally. He has one of those characters that fill you with passion. He certainly inspired me to change the way I viewed life and this change in my perception altered so much else.

— SIMON

Depression

Jerry Sargeant has helped me change my life in so many ways with his energy healing. Before I met Jerry I was in a very dark place – really suffering mentally. I felt so depressed and anxious that sometimes I couldn't even walk out of my front door. I was stuck on medication for ten years and felt like there was no hope.

Jerry then started to work with me and the results have been absolutely incredible. I am now medication free for the first time in ten years and I now feel happy and positive and I'm doing so many things now that I've never been able to do before. I've joined a walking group and am taking driving lessons.

Thank you Jerry from the bottom of my heart.

— LEIGH

Road Traffic Accident

I was riding my bicycle one day and as I approached a roundabout a car came across it. Both of us were going too fast. My head went straight through the tiny quarter light window. I pulled my head out and my face was hanging off. The next thing I remember was waking up in hospital.

My nose had been pushed into the back of my skull. My back and neck were broken and my face was torn to bits. The doctors didn't give me much hope. They cut the top of my head open, pulled my skull forward and pushed my nose back out. They stitched up my face and I was in intensive care.

I remember waking up and seeing what I can only describe as the devil waiting for me at the end of my bed. It was so vivid and real. My partner Karen got in touch with Jerry, and asked if he would do some healing. She could see that the drugs were not helping and the operations were not making me any better. She asked the doctors to stop trying out different drugs on me. It felt like I was an experiment.

I could feel one day that someone was touching me, on my head. I looked but no one was there. I then knew I was experiencing Jerry's

243

energy healing. I didn't believe in it before. But when I felt being touched and no one was there, I knew it was real.

Within twenty-four hours of the healing I could breathe normally and so I took the ventilator off. Within two weeks my face healed and the pain stopped. My back and neck just seemed to heal. I was back at work within weeks. The doctors could not believe the transformation.

When I went to see the doctors and had my back X-rayed it showed no signs of any damage. None at all. Just a few weeks before it showed major damage. It was as though the broken bones just fixed themselves. To go from being on death's door to back at work within five weeks is amazing. I am happy and living my life. I am very grateful that my partner found Jerry.

— STEPHAN

Anxiety

Before I met Jerry I was in a very dark place. I was suffering mild depression, struggling to deal with childhood experiences. I would suffer suicidal thoughts and voices in my head. It would go away for a while and then come back, and then in November last year it came back but even stronger. I was put on Anti-Depressants to help me get through. A few months later I realized that the medication wasn't helping me.

It made me feel tired and I didn't want to interact with anyone so I shut myself away. I was like a sponge to other people's negativity, which got me down, as well as my own life did and it got too much for me to cope with. Then I met Jerry. I received distance healing from Jerry and he put me on a diet and exercise plan. I soon felt great. I felt even better because I was 11st 3lbs in weight and within a few weeks I dropped to 9st 11lbs, something I wanted to do for a while. Since working with Jerry I have started to feel a lot better in my mind. The voices I had before have gone. I lost the will to live but now I want to live and am enjoying life a lot more. I feel like I have gone through a battle and through the other side. There are no words I can say to express how grateful I am for the help Jerry gave me. I am very grateful. Thank you Jerry, you gave me my life back.

— CHARLOTTE

Fibroids & Tumour

I was bleeding heavily and after going to the doctor discovered that I had fibroids and a Tumour in my uterus. I didn't want surgery so I looked for an alternative. I was searching for Psychic Surgeons in the Philippines and Jerry Sargeant popped up. I contacted Jerry and asked him for help.

Jerry did three healing sessions. I went back to the doctor and had scans a few weeks later. When my results came through the Fibroids were gone and so was the Tumour. It was a miracle. I am so grateful to Jerry for his help.

Thank You.

— MICKEY

Tumour

I had a tumour in my throat. After years of drug abuse, that had been triggered by a series of traumatic incidents in my life. My brother contacted Jerry and he came to my house, as he lived not too far away. I lay down and he did what he did. It was a beautiful experience, which lasted for two hours on and off.

I went to the doctor six weeks later and had some tests. The tumour (the size of a tomato) in my throat had disappeared. It was amazing. A miracle.

— ANDY

Haemorrhoids

When tough times came I would stress myself so hard, that I developed internal haemorrhoids and I would lose a lot of blood. Jerry and I talked about this and we agreed to do a distant healing. After relaxing on the bed I swear that I felt "someone" running inside me. A strange and funny sensation. Later I fell asleep. After only two sessions I felt much better. I was cured, no more haemorrhoids. The shifts were so powerful and strong, almost violent as Jerry was working on every cell within my soul. Questions of heart were so true and interesting at the same time. The fact that, in Jerry's words, "the heavy liquid black stuff" came out, was unknown to me, although I felt uneasiness for years.

What to say... Thank you, my dear Jerry.

— DANIEL

245

Love for the first time

Growing up in a family with lots of tension surrounding our ethnicity was very tough. Also, I didn't value myself and had no love for myself after a series of life events, including losing my own daughter to domestic violence. I decided to go to one of Jerry's workshop and then had a healing. During the healing Jerry took me into my childhood and showed me how to embrace my inner child. I regained my love for myself and increased my confidence.

My relationship with my children has gotten so much better since I reconnected with myself. I have had lots of healing before but they were surface level compared to Star Magic. Star Magic connected me in a way I've never been connected before. I could feel all of my barriers come down during the healing. I let go and everything released. Jerry created the environment so I could do that. It was a big achievement for me. I am so grateful.

— LAVENDER

Symbol for Charging
Water with Love

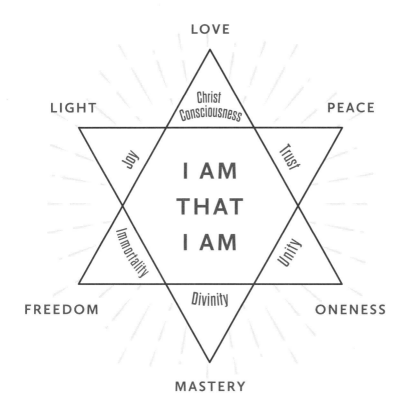

Symbol for charging water with love

This symbol will change the molecular structure of your water, dissolve the fluoride and other chemicals in it, and charge it with love. Please cut out or photocopy this symbol several times and stick it to bottles with filtered water. Leave the water to sit for two days before using it.

Illustration Guide

Index

About the Author

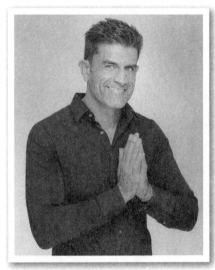

Photo by Larisa Dizdar

JERRY SARGEANT known as "The Facilitator", is the founder of Star Magic Healing. He is world renowned for healing people and creating rapid shifts within them on the mental, physical, emotional and spiritual plane. Jerry's mission is to set the human race free by expanding consciousness on Planet Earth through the Star Magic Matrix, a powerful energetic grid of light that is being constructed around our planet.

Jerry knows about setting one's self free. Being a drug addict from a young age and walking a different path, which led to mixing with some of the world's most dangerous criminals, Jerry broke free from this life after a number of life-altering events. A near fatal car crash, a trip to Alpha Centauri in a space craft, an encounter with an Angel and time spent in Egyptian Mystery Schools underneath the Great Pyramids, led him to insights and precious information enabling him to access and harness super-transformative healing energy.

Jerry's ability to heal has been likened to some of the most powerful healers in history, having healed broken bones, removed tumours, cysts, dissolved fibromyalgia, healed hearts as well as healing broken relationships and super-charging businesses to achieve massive success.

Star Magic, as well as being the most powerful healing modality on the planet, is a lifestyle. It's an opportunity to be free, mentally, physically, emotionally and spiritually. It's a way of being free to do what you want, when you want, with whomever you want, for as long as you want. Star Magic is a way of life, a lifestyle that you will live with passion, once you harness and know the power that lies within your own genetic make-up. Star Magic is the key to unlock the door to a free, loving and compassionate world. A space nurtured and cradled in love.

Jerry's vision is to harness extra-terrestrial light frequencies and bring them safely and effectively to Planet Earth, through a number of Star Magic Healing Facilities, strategically placed around the Christ Consciousness Grid of our planet. The codes contained within the light will elevate consciousness in a phenomenal way and create freedom for human-kind, by connecting every man, woman and child, through their heart, to unconditional love.

Jerry runs a number of Star Magic healing and meditation workshops, a Global Meditation Group and trains people to create with Star Magic and work with the light and sound codes, constantly travelling through the ether. You can find out more about Jerry and his work with Star Magic here: **www.starmagichealing.com**

Jerry is available for speaking engagements worldwide. If you would like Jerry to speak at your event, please contact **info@starmagichealing.com**

Star Magic Academy

Do you feel a pull inside of you? A calling? Something deep that is yearning for more? Abundance in all areas of your life? A deep desire to assist in the growth of humanity? The Star Magic Academy offers you the opportunity to realize your full potential, in this reality. Whether you are an experienced healer, a total beginner or a woman or man on a mission, wanting to add serious value to this Planet and assist in guiding your fellow sisters and brothers, your human family, on their journey to freedom where a high-vibrational experience is created for everyone, then you've found your way home.

Vision

Our vision is to build healing centres in strategic locations around the Planet and to train dedicated people to work with us, inside these centres, side by side, to elevate the frequency of our human family and Mother Earth herself.

Once trained you will live a Star Magic Life Style, travelling, facilitating healing, running workshops and trainings to further expand and share the Star Magic Frequency, so everyone can shift and expand their consciousness in an accelerated fashion, connected on the frequency of unconditional love, united as one Universal Force, through Star Magic.

The Academy

Firstly, this isn't for the faint-hearted. It is for those human beings that truly want to thrive in this world and live 24/7 in a state of elevated vibration.

You will be guided by Jerry and the Star Magic team through a multi-layered process, spanning four levels. Level one is the Facilitator Training. Level two is the Advanced Frequency Upgrade. Level three is Through the Star Gate. Level four is the Master Facilitator.

As you complete each training you will be asked to come back and assist in future trainings and help with the facilitation. This, amongst other tasks, will get you your Stars. Once you accumulate a specific number of Stars at each Frequency Band (level in your training), you will move up to the next Frequency Band and continue on your journey to being a Master Facilitator.

For more information on Star Magic Workshops and Training Experiences please visit **www.starmagichealing.com**

The Star Magic Tribe is Your Tribe
We welcome you with a fearless open heart

Also of interest from Findhorn Press

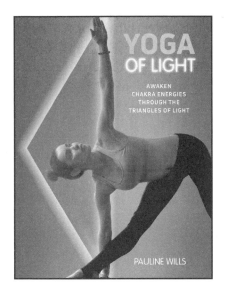

Yoga of Light

by Pauline Wills

DRAWING ON YOGA'S ORIGINAL TEACHINGS, Pauline
Wills reveals how to awaken and energize the chakra triangles of
light with the practice of yoga asanas, breathing, visualization,
and meditation. Includes an illustrated step-by-step guide to
performing the asanas correctly and depicts the triangles of light
formed by each and their specific health benefits.

ISBN 9-781-62055-944-4

FINDHORN PRESS

Life-Changing Books

Learn more about us and our books at:
www.findhornpress.com

For information on the Findhorn Foundation:
www.findhorn.org